THIS PLANNER BELONGS TO

NAME: SARAH JEAN

PHONE: 330-391-1005

E-MAIL: SARAH@LOSERFACE.COM

THE JOURNEY BEGINS

before

CHEST

WAIST

HIPS

THIGHS

after

CHEST

WAIST

HIPS

THIGHS

MEASUREMENTS

BEFORE	AFTER
DRESS SIZE	DRESS SIZE
CHEST	CHEST
ARMS	ARMS
WAIST	WAIST
HIPS	HIPS
THIGHS	THIGHS
WEIGHT	WEIGHT

FITNESS HEALTH TIPS

- Drink enough water and try to avoid sugary drinks/sodas!

- Sleep between 7-9 hours each day. Lost sleep can't be compensated, thus creating a balanced lifestyle is your best choice.

- Try meditation, there is nothing better for achieving your fitness&diet goals than a strong mind.

- Exercise daily - pick activities that you enjoy doing, this way it will be much easier to be consistent.

- Workout all parts of your body, don't focus on a sport or activity that only trains your legs, go for a variety of activities that will train your whole body.

- Eat more fruits and vegetables. They are not only healthy, but also contain fewer calories and make you feel sated.

- Go for a long everyday. You can listen to an audiobook while doing this. This way you will not only lose weight, but gain knowledge at the same time.

- Clean your kitchen from all sweet and processed foods. Not looking the temptation in the eye is the best way to avoid it.

- Avoid alcohol and smoking at all costs, no need to explain how bad they are for your body.

- Love yourself - no matter where you begin your journey perfection is not the end goal, but to get better everyday.

- Nothing feels as fulfilling as making progress towards your goals!

CALCULATING YOUR DESIRED CALORIC INTAKE

In order to lose weight the most important step is to know how much calories you need in a day. And how much you need to consume to lose weight. This will be your target. So first let's establish your Basal Metabolic Rate (**BMR**)

For Women: **BMR** = 665 + (4.35 x W) + (4.7 x H) - (4.7 x A)
For Men: **BMR** = 66 + (6.23 x W) + (12.7 x H) - (6.8 x A)

Where **W** is your weights in pounds, **H** is your height in inches and **A** is your age.

Once you have your **BMR** the next step is to multiply it based on your activity level:
Sedentary (No sports activity at all) **x1.2**
Lightly active (doing sports 1-2 times a week) **x1.375**
Moderately active (3-5 times a week) **x1.55**
Very active (doing sports daily) **x1.725**

Now you have you calorie intake for the day. With this calorie intake you are going to maintain your weight. if you want to lose weight, you have to reduce the calories in order to create a caloric deficit.
You can do this by multiplying your calorie intake that you have calculated above. This way you can achieve various levels of weight loss depending on your goals:
For **mild weight loss** multiply your calorie intake by **x0.9** this way you will lose **0.5lb/week**
For **moderate weight loss** multiply your calorie intake by **x0.8** this way you will lose **1lb/week**
For **extreme weight loss** multiply your calorie intake by **x0.675** this way you will lose **1.5lb/week***

EXAMPLE:

If you are a woman with weight **W=150lb**, height **H=65in** and if your age **A=30** years old, then your
BMR = 665 + (4.35 x 150) + (4.7 x 65) - (4.7 x 30) = 1,472 kcal/day
If you have a ightly avtive livestyle, then your total calorie intake should be: **BMR x 1.375** = 1,472 x 1,375 = **2024 kcal**
This is the calories you should consume in order to maintain your weight. If you want to lose weight, for example 1lb/week you should multiply 2024x0.8 = **1619,2 ckal** with this caloric intake you will be able to lose weight at a steady pace.

Calculate your BMR and Caloric intake:**
W =
H =
A =
BMR = 66 + (6.23 x   ) + (12.7 x   ) - (6.8 x   ) =

Multiply it by your activity level and then by your
desired weight loss goal.

MY DESIRED CALORIE INTAKE:
- -

*If you plan to do extreme weight loss, please consult with your doctor first!
** You have more space to make calculations and notes at the end of this planner

CALORIE CALCULATOR

MODERATE PHYSICAL ACTIVITIES	IN 1 HOUR	IN 30 MINUTES
Hiking	370	185
Light gardening / yard work	330	165
Dancing	330	165
Golf (walking and carrying clubs)	330	165
Bicycling (less than 10 mph)	290	145
Walking (3.5 mph)	280	140
Weight Training (general light workout)	220	110
Streching	180	90
VIGOROUS PHYSICAL ACTIVITIES	**IN 1 HOUR**	**IN 30 MINUTES**
Running / Jogging (5 mph)	590	295
Bicycling (more than 10 mph)	590	295
Swimming (slow freestyle laps)	510	255
Aerobics	480	240
Walking (4.5 mph)	460	230
Heavy yard work (chopping wood)	440	220
Weight lifting (vigorous effort)	440	220
Basketball (vigorous)	440	220

TYPE	QUANTITY	CALORIES
Full-fat milk	1 cup	150
Low fat milk (1%)	1 cup	102
Cow's milk	1 cup	157
Goat milk	1 cup	264
Sweetened Condensed Milk "cans"	1oz	123
Full cream milk powder	Half a cup	635
Cheddar cheese slices	Slice, 1oz	114
Feta cheese	1oz	75
Finuta cheese	1oz	110
Gouda cheese	1oz	101
Mozzarella cheese	1oz	80
Kraft Cheese "cups"	1oz	80
Edam cheese	1oz	98
Blue cheese	1oz	104
Mascarpone cheese	1oz	128
Ricotta cheese "whole milk"	Half a cup	216
Parmesan cheese	1oz	130
Camembert cheese	1oz	86
Cottage cheese	3.5oz	99
Halloumi cheese	3.5oz	363
ICE CREAM		
Vanilla	1 ball	240
Cocoa	1 ball	280
Strawberries		220
DRINKS & JUICES		
Apple juice	Half a cup	60
Apricot juice, canned	Half a cup	72
Grape juice, canned	Half a cup	78
Fresh orange juice	Half a cup	59
Canned orange juice	Half a cup	52
Grapefruit juice, canned local	Half a cup	58
Grapefruit juice, unsweetened	Half a cup	47

TYPE	QUANTITY	CALORIES
Canned peach juice	Half a cup	67
Canned pear juice	Half a cup	75
Canned pineapple juice	Half a cup	70
Canned tomato juice	Half a cup	21
EGGS		
Egg whites, (fresh or iced)	One, big	17
Fresh egg yolk	One, big	59
Full cook boiled eggs	One, big	79
Fried eggs	One, big	91
Omelet with cheese and vegetables	4oz	252
NUTS & LEGUMES		
Nuts	Half a cup, 2.5oz	380
Almonds, dry	Quarter a cup	209
Cashew, roasted, dry	1oz	160
Nuts, roasted, dry	1oz	170
Hazelnut, roasted, oily	1oz	176
Lentils, whole, green	Half a cup	215
OILS & FATS		
Olive oil	1 Tablespoon	120
Sunflower oil	1 Tablespoon	120
Vegetable oil	1 Tablespoon	126
Butter	1 Tablespoon	36
Cocoa	1 ball	280
RED MEAT		
Lamb thigh, roasted without fat	3oz	140
Lamb rib, grilled without fat	3oz	200
Pork	3oz	202
Beef, chest, cooked	3oz	189
Beef shoulder, without fat	3oz	183
Beef, minced and cooked	3oz	245
Beef steak without fat	3oz	174
Kebab	3oz	226

TYPE	QUANTITY	CALORIES
FRESH FRUITS		
Apples	Medium, 4.5oz	81
Apricot	Medium, 1oz	17
Banana	Medium, 3.5oz	105
Fig	One, 40 g	37
Grapefruit	Half	38
Cherries	10 beads	49
Avocado	Half	162
Grapes	Half a cup	53
Guava	One, 3oz	45
Kiwi	One, 2.5oz	46
Mango	Half, 3oz	68
Orange	One, 3.75oz	62
Papaya	Medium	117
Peach	One, 3oz	37
Pear	Medium, 6oz	98
Pineapple	Slice, 3oz	42
Plum	One, 2oz	36
Pomegranate	Medium, 5oz	110
Nectarine	Medium, 5oz	67
Watermelon	Piece, 3.5oz	26
Melon	Piece, 3.5oz	33
Strawberries	Half a cup	23
Tangerine	One, 3oz	37
Blueberry	One cup	122
Rutab/ripe dates	10 beads	150
Loquat	3.5oz	49
Plum	3.5oz	52
Lemon	3.5oz	17
Sweet Lemon	Fruit size	53
Black berry	One cup	117
Nabq (rhamnus)	30 beads	9
Quince	Medium	60

TYPE	QUANTITY	CALORIES
Tamarind	Half a cup	82
VEGETABLES		
Carrot	Medium, 2.5oz	31
Cauliflower, cooked	Half a cup	15
Cucumbers, chopped	Half a cup	7
Eggplant, cooked	Half a cup	13
Green beans, cooked	Half a cup	20
Cabbage, cooked	Half a cup	16
Celery	Half a cup	10
Corn	One, medium	77
Mushrooms, fresh	Half a cup	9
Lettuce	Half a cup	4
Fresh onions, chopped	Half a cup	27
Green onions, chopped	Half a cup	16
Green peas, cooked	Half a cup	67
Peppers, chopped	Half a cup	12
Hot pepper	One, 1oz	18
Baked potato, with the peel	7oz	220
Fried potato	10 pieces, 1.5oz	158
Shalgam kale, boiled	Half a cup	14
Squash	Half a cup	41
Chopped spinach	Half a cup	6
Sweet potatoes, mashed	Piece, 3.5oz	33
Red tomatoes	Half a cup	111
Green beans	One cup	73
Beet	One cup	46
Cabbage	One cup	73
Leek	1 Spoon, minced	1
Black olives	10 grains, medium	95
Green olives	10 grains, medium	66
Parsley	Package, medium	25
Spinach	1 Cup, chopped	14
Zucchini	1 Cup, chopped	31
Sugar-cane	3.5oz	82

PROGRESS TRACKER

WEEK 1	1	2	3	4	5	6	7	WEEK 27	183	184	185	186	187	188	189
WEEK 2	8	9	10	11	12	13	14	WEEK 28	190	191	192	193	194	195	196
WEEK 3	15	16	17	18	19	20	21	WEEK 29	197	198	199	200	201	202	203
WEEK 4	22	23	24	25	26	27	28	WEEK 30	204	205	206	207	208	209	210
WEEK 5	29	30	31	32	33	34	35	WEEK 31	211	212	213	214	215	216	217
WEEK 6	36	37	38	39	40	41	42	WEEK 32	218	219	220	221	222	223	224
WEEK 7	43	44	45	46	47	48	49	WEEK 33	225	226	227	228	229	230	231
WEEK 8	50	51	52	53	54	55	56	WEEK 34	232	233	234	235	236	237	238
WEEK 9	57	58	59	60	61	62	63	WEEK 35	239	240	241	242	243	244	245
WEEK 10	64	65	66	67	68	69	70	WEEK 36	246	247	248	249	250	251	252
WEEK 11	71	72	73	74	75	76	77	WEEK 37	253	254	255	256	257	258	259
WEEK 12	78	79	80	81	82	83	84	WEEK 38	260	261	262	263	264	265	266
WEEK 13	85	86	87	88	89	90	91	WEEK 39	267	268	269	270	271	272	273
WEEK 14	92	93	94	95	96	97	98	WEEK 40	274	275	276	277	278	279	280
WEEK 15	99	100	101	102	103	104	105	WEEK 41	281	282	283	284	285	286	287
WEEK 16	106	107	108	109	110	111	112	WEEK 42	288	289	290	291	292	293	294
WEEK 17	113	114	115	116	117	118	119	WEEK 43	295	296	297	298	299	300	301
WEEK 18	120	121	122	123	124	125	126	WEEK 44	302	303	304	305	306	307	308
WEEK 19	127	128	129	130	131	132	133	WEEK 45	309	310	311	312	313	314	315
WEEK 20	134	135	136	137	138	139	140	WEEK 46	316	317	318	320	321	322	323
WEEK 21	141	142	143	144	145	146	147	WEEK 47	324	325	326	327	328	329	330
WEEK 22	148	149	150	151	152	153	154	WEEK 48	331	332	333	334	335	336	337
WEEK 23	155	156	157	158	159	160	161	WEEK 49	338	339	340	341	342	343	344
WEEK 24	162	163	164	165	166	167	168	WEEK 50	345	346	347	348	349	350	351
WEEK 25	169	170	171	172	173	174	175	WEEK 51	352	353	354	355	356	357
WEEK 26	176	177	178	179	180	181	182	WEEK 52	358	359	360	361	362	363	364

HOW TO FILL YOUR FITNESS PLANNER

WEEK #1

Write down what you eat during each day

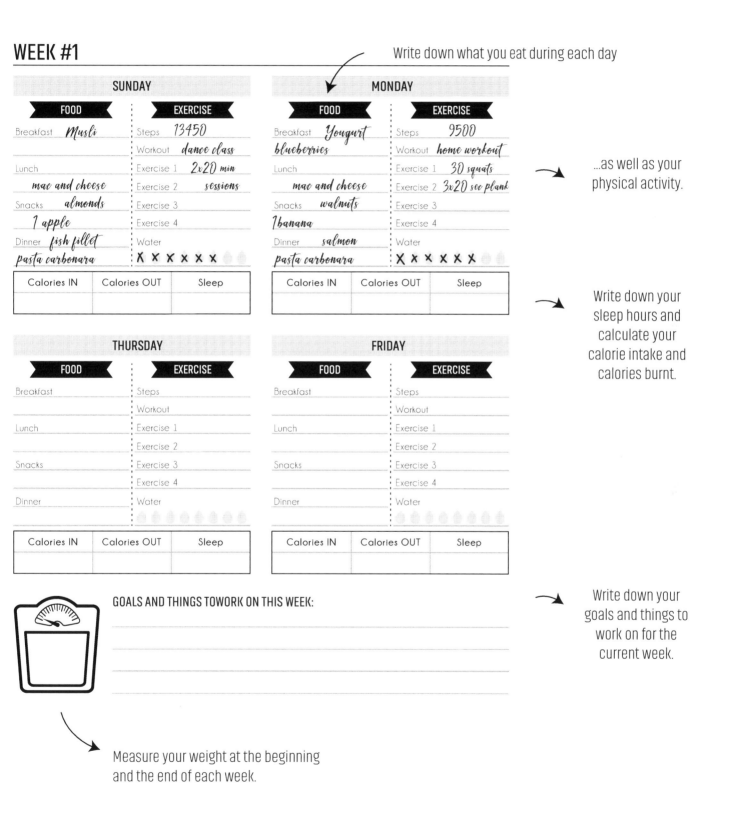

SUNDAY

FOOD	EXERCISE
Breakfast *Musli*	Steps *13450*
	Workout *dance class*
Lunch	Exercise 1 *2x20 min*
mac and cheese	Exercise 2 *sessions*
Snacks *almonds*	Exercise 3
1 apple	Exercise 4
Dinner *fish fillet*	Water
pasta carbonara	X X X X X

Calories IN	Calories OUT	Sleep

MONDAY

FOOD	EXERCISE
Breakfast *Yougurt*	Steps *9500*
blueberries	Workout *home workout*
Lunch	Exercise 1 *30 squats*
mac and cheese	Exercise 2 *3x20 sec plank*
Snacks *walnuts*	Exercise 3
1 banana	Exercise 4
Dinner *salmon*	Water
pasta carbonara	X X X X X

Calories IN	Calories OUT	Sleep

...as well as your physical activity.

Write down your sleep hours and calculate your calorie intake and calories burnt.

THURSDAY

FOOD	EXERCISE
Breakfast	Steps
	Workout
Lunch	Exercise 1
	Exercise 2
Snacks	Exercise 3
	Exercise 4
Dinner	Water

Calories IN	Calories OUT	Sleep

FRIDAY

FOOD	EXERCISE
Breakfast	Steps
	Workout
Lunch	Exercise 1
	Exercise 2
Snacks	Exercise 3
	Exercise 4
Dinner	Water

Calories IN	Calories OUT	Sleep

GOALS AND THINGS TO WORK ON THIS WEEK:

Write down your goals and things to work on for the current week.

Measure your weight at the beginning and the end of each week.

WEEK #1

SUNDAY

FOOD

Breakfast

Lunch

Snacks

Dinner

EXERCISE

Steps

Workout

Exercise 1

Exercise 2

Exercise 3

Exercise 4

Water

Calories IN	Calories OUT	Sleep

MONDAY

FOOD

Breakfast

Lunch

Snacks

Dinner

EXERCISE

Steps

Workout

Exercise 1

Exercise 2

Exercise 3

Exercise 4

Water

Calories IN	Calories OUT	Sleep

THURSDAY

FOOD

Breakfast

Lunch

Snacks

Dinner

EXERCISE

Steps

Workout

Exercise 1

Exercise 2

Exercise 3

Exercise 4

Water

Calories IN	Calories OUT	Sleep

FRIDAY

FOOD

Breakfast

Lunch

Snacks

Dinner

EXERCISE

Steps

Workout

Exercise 1

Exercise 2

Exercise 3

Exercise 4

Water

Calories IN	Calories OUT	Sleep

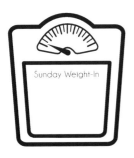

Sunday Weight-In

GOALS AND THINGS TO WORK ON THIS WEEK:

TUESDAY

FOOD

Breakfast

Lunch

Snacks

Dinner

EXERCISE

Steps

Workout

Exercise 1

Exercise 2

Exercise 3

Exercise 4

Water

Calories IN	Calories OUT	Sleep

WEDNESDAY

FOOD

Breakfast

Lunch

Snacks

Dinner

EXERCISE

Steps

Workout

Exercise 1

Exercise 2

Exercise 3

Exercise 4

Water

Calories IN	Calories OUT	Sleep

SATURDAY

FOOD

Breakfast

Lunch

Snacks

Dinner

EXERCISE

Steps

Workout

Exercise 1

Exercise 2

Exercise 3

Exercise 4

Water

Calories IN	Calories OUT	Sleep

WEEKLY SUMMARY

WORKOUTS THIS WEEK

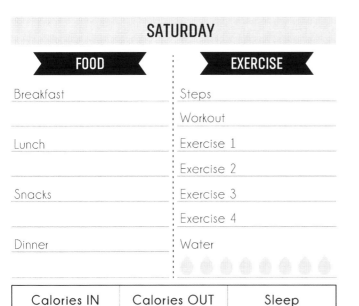

HOW HAPPY ARE YOU WITH YOUR PROGRESS

AVERAGE WATER

Calories IN	Calories OUT	Sleep

GOALS AND THINGS TO WORK ON THIS WEEK:

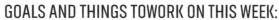

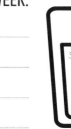

Saturday Weight-In

WEEK #2

SUNDAY

FOOD
Breakfast

Lunch

Snacks

Dinner

EXERCISE
Steps

Workout

Exercise 1

Exercise 2

Exercise 3

Exercise 4

Water

Calories IN	Calories OUT	Sleep

MONDAY

FOOD
Breakfast

Lunch

Snacks

Dinner

EXERCISE
Steps

Workout

Exercise 1

Exercise 2

Exercise 3

Exercise 4

Water

Calories IN	Calories OUT	Sleep

THURSDAY

FOOD
Breakfast

Lunch

Snacks

Dinner

EXERCISE
Steps

Workout

Exercise 1

Exercise 2

Exercise 3

Exercise 4

Water

Calories IN	Calories OUT	Sleep

FRIDAY

FOOD
Breakfast

Lunch

Snacks

Dinner

EXERCISE
Steps

Workout

Exercise 1

Exercise 2

Exercise 3

Exercise 4

Water

Calories IN	Calories OUT	Sleep

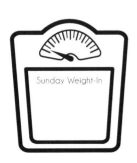

Sunday Weight-In

GOALS AND THINGS TO WORK ON THIS WEEK:

TUESDAY

FOOD

Breakfast

Lunch

Snacks

Dinner

EXERCISE

Steps

Workout

Exercise 1

Exercise 2

Exercise 3

Exercise 4

Water

Calories IN	Calories OUT	Sleep

WEDNESDAY

FOOD

Breakfast

Lunch

Snacks

Dinner

EXERCISE

Steps

Workout

Exercise 1

Exercise 2

Exercise 3

Exercise 4

Water

Calories IN	Calories OUT	Sleep

SATURDAY

FOOD

Breakfast

Lunch

Snacks

Dinner

EXERCISE

Steps

Workout

Exercise 1

Exercise 2

Exercise 3

Exercise 4

Water

Calories IN	Calories OUT	Sleep

WEEKLY SUMMARY

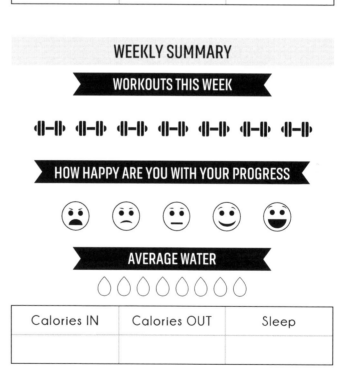

WORKOUTS THIS WEEK

HOW HAPPY ARE YOU WITH YOUR PROGRESS

AVERAGE WATER

Calories IN	Calories OUT	Sleep

GOALS AND THINGS TO WORK ON THIS WEEK:

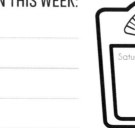

Saturday Weight-In

WEEK #3

SUNDAY

FOOD

Breakfast

Lunch

Snacks

Dinner

EXERCISE

Steps

Workout

Exercise 1

Exercise 2

Exercise 3

Exercise 4

Water

Calories IN	Calories OUT	Sleep

MONDAY

FOOD

Breakfast

Lunch

Snacks

Dinner

EXERCISE

Steps

Workout

Exercise 1

Exercise 2

Exercise 3

Exercise 4

Water

Calories IN	Calories OUT	Sleep

THURSDAY

FOOD

Breakfast

Lunch

Snacks

Dinner

EXERCISE

Steps

Workout

Exercise 1

Exercise 2

Exercise 3

Exercise 4

Water

Calories IN	Calories OUT	Sleep

FRIDAY

FOOD

Breakfast

Lunch

Snacks

Dinner

EXERCISE

Steps

Workout

Exercise 1

Exercise 2

Exercise 3

Exercise 4

Water

Calories IN	Calories OUT	Sleep

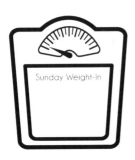

Sunday Weight-In

GOALS AND THINGS TO WORK ON THIS WEEK:

TUESDAY

FOOD

Breakfast

Lunch

Snacks

Dinner

EXERCISE

Steps

Workout

Exercise 1

Exercise 2

Exercise 3

Exercise 4

Water

Calories IN	Calories OUT	Sleep

WEDNESDAY

FOOD

Breakfast

Lunch

Snacks

Dinner

EXERCISE

Steps

Workout

Exercise 1

Exercise 2

Exercise 3

Exercise 4

Water

Calories IN	Calories OUT	Sleep

SATURDAY

FOOD

Breakfast

Lunch

Snacks

Dinner

EXERCISE

Steps

Workout

Exercise 1

Exercise 2

Exercise 3

Exercise 4

Water

Calories IN	Calories OUT	Sleep

WEEKLY SUMMARY

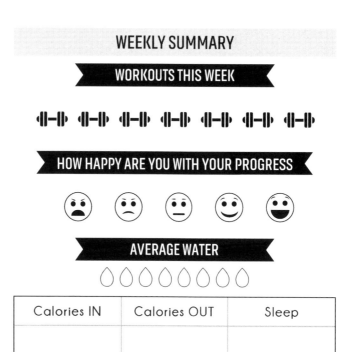

WORKOUTS THIS WEEK

HOW HAPPY ARE YOU WITH YOUR PROGRESS

AVERAGE WATER

Calories IN	Calories OUT	Sleep

GOALS AND THINGS TO WORK ON THIS WEEK:

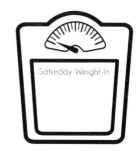

Saturday Weight-In

WEEK #4

SUNDAY

FOOD

Breakfast

Lunch

Snacks

Dinner

EXERCISE

Steps

Workout

Exercise 1

Exercise 2

Exercise 3

Exercise 4

Water

Calories IN	Calories OUT	Sleep

MONDAY

FOOD

Breakfast

Lunch

Snacks

Dinner

EXERCISE

Steps

Workout

Exercise 1

Exercise 2

Exercise 3

Exercise 4

Water

Calories IN	Calories OUT	Sleep

THURSDAY

FOOD

Breakfast

Lunch

Snacks

Dinner

EXERCISE

Steps

Workout

Exercise 1

Exercise 2

Exercise 3

Exercise 4

Water

Calories IN	Calories OUT	Sleep

FRIDAY

FOOD

Breakfast

Lunch

Snacks

Dinner

EXERCISE

Steps

Workout

Exercise 1

Exercise 2

Exercise 3

Exercise 4

Water

Calories IN	Calories OUT	Sleep

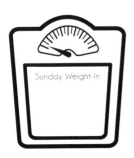

Sunday Weight-In

GOALS AND THINGS TO WORK ON THIS WEEK:

TUESDAY

FOOD

Breakfast

Lunch

Snacks

Dinner

EXERCISE

Steps

Workout

Exercise 1

Exercise 2

Exercise 3

Exercise 4

Water

Calories IN	Calories OUT	Sleep

WEDNESDAY

FOOD

Breakfast

Lunch

Snacks

Dinner

EXERCISE

Steps

Workout

Exercise 1

Exercise 2

Exercise 3

Exercise 4

Water

Calories IN	Calories OUT	Sleep

SATURDAY

FOOD

Breakfast

Lunch

Snacks

Dinner

EXERCISE

Steps

Workout

Exercise 1

Exercise 2

Exercise 3

Exercise 4

Water

Calories IN	Calories OUT	Sleep

WEEKLY SUMMARY

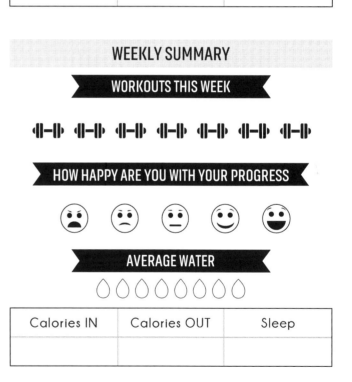

WORKOUTS THIS WEEK

HOW HAPPY ARE YOU WITH YOUR PROGRESS

AVERAGE WATER

Calories IN	Calories OUT	Sleep

GOALS AND THINGS TO WORK ON THIS WEEK:

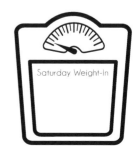

Saturday Weight-In

WEEK #5

SUNDAY

FOOD

Breakfast

Lunch

Snacks

Dinner

EXERCISE

Steps

Workout

Exercise 1

Exercise 2

Exercise 3

Exercise 4

Water

Calories IN	Calories OUT	Sleep

MONDAY

FOOD

Breakfast

Lunch

Snacks

Dinner

EXERCISE

Steps

Workout

Exercise 1

Exercise 2

Exercise 3

Exercise 4

Water

Calories IN	Calories OUT	Sleep

THURSDAY

FOOD

Breakfast

Lunch

Snacks

Dinner

EXERCISE

Steps

Workout

Exercise 1

Exercise 2

Exercise 3

Exercise 4

Water

Calories IN	Calories OUT	Sleep

FRIDAY

FOOD

Breakfast

Lunch

Snacks

Dinner

EXERCISE

Steps

Workout

Exercise 1

Exercise 2

Exercise 3

Exercise 4

Water

Calories IN	Calories OUT	Sleep

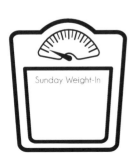

Sunday Weight-In

GOALS AND THINGS TO WORK ON THIS WEEK:

TUESDAY

FOOD

Breakfast

Lunch

Snacks

Dinner

EXERCISE

Steps

Workout

Exercise 1

Exercise 2

Exercise 3

Exercise 4

Water

Calories IN	Calories OUT	Sleep

WEDNESDAY

FOOD

Breakfast

Lunch

Snacks

Dinner

EXERCISE

Steps

Workout

Exercise 1

Exercise 2

Exercise 3

Exercise 4

Water

Calories IN	Calories OUT	Sleep

SATURDAY

FOOD

Breakfast

Lunch

Snacks

Dinner

EXERCISE

Steps

Workout

Exercise 1

Exercise 2

Exercise 3

Exercise 4

Water

Calories IN	Calories OUT	Sleep

WEEKLY SUMMARY

WORKOUTS THIS WEEK

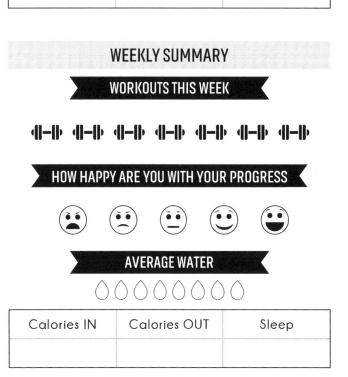

HOW HAPPY ARE YOU WITH YOUR PROGRESS

AVERAGE WATER

Calories IN	Calories OUT	Sleep

GOALS AND THINGS TO WORK ON THIS WEEK:

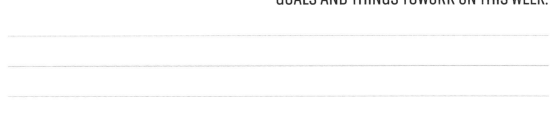

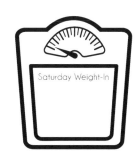

Saturday Weight-In

WEEK #6

SUNDAY

FOOD	EXERCISE
Breakfast	Steps
	Workout
Lunch	Exercise 1
	Exercise 2
Snacks	Exercise 3
	Exercise 4
Dinner	Water

Calories IN	Calories OUT	Sleep

MONDAY

FOOD	EXERCISE
Breakfast	Steps
	Workout
Lunch	Exercise 1
	Exercise 2
Snacks	Exercise 3
	Exercise 4
Dinner	Water

Calories IN	Calories OUT	Sleep

THURSDAY

FOOD	EXERCISE
Breakfast	Steps
	Workout
Lunch	Exercise 1
	Exercise 2
Snacks	Exercise 3
	Exercise 4
Dinner	Water

Calories IN	Calories OUT	Sleep

FRIDAY

FOOD	EXERCISE
Breakfast	Steps
	Workout
Lunch	Exercise 1
	Exercise 2
Snacks	Exercise 3
	Exercise 4
Dinner	Water

Calories IN	Calories OUT	Sleep

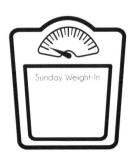

Sunday Weight-In

GOALS AND THINGS TO WORK ON THIS WEEK:

TUESDAY

FOOD

Breakfast

Lunch

Snacks

Dinner

EXERCISE

Steps

Workout

Exercise 1

Exercise 2

Exercise 3

Exercise 4

Water

Calories IN	Calories OUT	Sleep

WEDNESDAY

FOOD

Breakfast

Lunch

Snacks

Dinner

EXERCISE

Steps

Workout

Exercise 1

Exercise 2

Exercise 3

Exercise 4

Water

Calories IN	Calories OUT	Sleep

SATURDAY

FOOD

Breakfast

Lunch

Snacks

Dinner

EXERCISE

Steps

Workout

Exercise 1

Exercise 2

Exercise 3

Exercise 4

Water

Calories IN	Calories OUT	Sleep

WEEKLY SUMMARY

WORKOUTS THIS WEEK

HOW HAPPY ARE YOU WITH YOUR PROGRESS

AVERAGE WATER

Calories IN	Calories OUT	Sleep

GOALS AND THINGS TO WORK ON THIS WEEK:

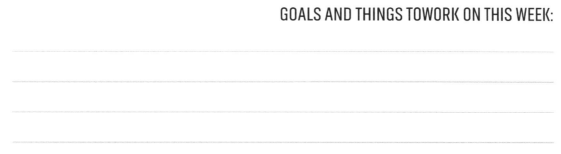

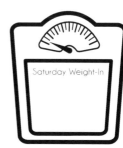

Saturday Weight-In

WEEK #7

SUNDAY

FOOD	EXERCISE
Breakfast	Steps
	Workout
Lunch	Exercise 1
	Exercise 2
Snacks	Exercise 3
	Exercise 4
Dinner	Water

Calories IN	Calories OUT	Sleep

MONDAY

FOOD	EXERCISE
Breakfast	Steps
	Workout
Lunch	Exercise 1
	Exercise 2
Snacks	Exercise 3
	Exercise 4
Dinner	Water

Calories IN	Calories OUT	Sleep

THURSDAY

FOOD	EXERCISE
Breakfast	Steps
	Workout
Lunch	Exercise 1
	Exercise 2
Snacks	Exercise 3
	Exercise 4
Dinner	Water

Calories IN	Calories OUT	Sleep

FRIDAY

FOOD	EXERCISE
Breakfast	Steps
	Workout
Lunch	Exercise 1
	Exercise 2
Snacks	Exercise 3
	Exercise 4
Dinner	Water

Calories IN	Calories OUT	Sleep

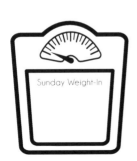

Sunday Weight-In

GOALS AND THINGS TO WORK ON THIS WEEK:

WEEK #7

TUESDAY

FOOD

Breakfast

Lunch

Snacks

Dinner

EXERCISE

Steps

Workout

Exercise 1

Exercise 2

Exercise 3

Exercise 4

Water

Calories IN	Calories OUT	Sleep

WEDNESDAY

FOOD

Breakfast

Lunch

Snacks

Dinner

EXERCISE

Steps

Workout

Exercise 1

Exercise 2

Exercise 3

Exercise 4

Water

Calories IN	Calories OUT	Sleep

SATURDAY

FOOD

Breakfast

Lunch

Snacks

Dinner

EXERCISE

Steps

Workout

Exercise 1

Exercise 2

Exercise 3

Exercise 4

Water

Calories IN	Calories OUT	Sleep

WEEKLY SUMMARY

WORKOUTS THIS WEEK

HOW HAPPY ARE YOU WITH YOUR PROGRESS

AVERAGE WATER

Calories IN	Calories OUT	Sleep

GOALS AND THINGS TO WORK ON THIS WEEK:

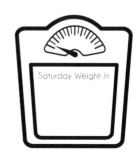

Saturday Weight-In

WEEK #8

SUNDAY

FOOD
Breakfast

Lunch

Snacks

Dinner

EXERCISE
Steps

Workout

Exercise 1

Exercise 2

Exercise 3

Exercise 4

Water

Calories IN	Calories OUT	Sleep

MONDAY

FOOD
Breakfast

Lunch

Snacks

Dinner

EXERCISE
Steps

Workout

Exercise 1

Exercise 2

Exercise 3

Exercise 4

Water

Calories IN	Calories OUT	Sleep

THURSDAY

FOOD
Breakfast

Lunch

Snacks

Dinner

EXERCISE
Steps

Workout

Exercise 1

Exercise 2

Exercise 3

Exercise 4

Water

Calories IN	Calories OUT	Sleep

FRIDAY

FOOD
Breakfast

Lunch

Snacks

Dinner

EXERCISE
Steps

Workout

Exercise 1

Exercise 2

Exercise 3

Exercise 4

Water

Calories IN	Calories OUT	Sleep

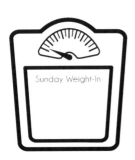

Sunday Weight-In

GOALS AND THINGS TO WORK ON THIS WEEK:

TUESDAY

FOOD

Breakfast

Lunch

Snacks

Dinner

EXERCISE

Steps

Workout

Exercise 1

Exercise 2

Exercise 3

Exercise 4

Water

Calories IN	Calories OUT	Sleep

WEDNESDAY

FOOD

Breakfast

Lunch

Snacks

Dinner

EXERCISE

Steps

Workout

Exercise 1

Exercise 2

Exercise 3

Exercise 4

Water

Calories IN	Calories OUT	Sleep

SATURDAY

FOOD

Breakfast

Lunch

Snacks

Dinner

EXERCISE

Steps

Workout

Exercise 1

Exercise 2

Exercise 3

Exercise 4

Water

Calories IN	Calories OUT	Sleep

WEEKLY SUMMARY

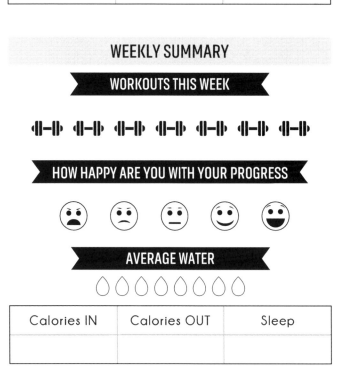

WORKOUTS THIS WEEK

HOW HAPPY ARE YOU WITH YOUR PROGRESS

AVERAGE WATER

Calories IN	Calories OUT	Sleep

GOALS AND THINGS TOWORK ON THIS WEEK:

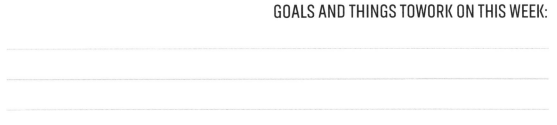

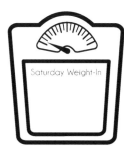

Saturday Weight-In

WEEK #9

SUNDAY

FOOD
Breakfast

Lunch

Snacks

Dinner

EXERCISE
Steps

Workout

Exercise 1

Exercise 2

Exercise 3

Exercise 4

Water

Calories IN	Calories OUT	Sleep

MONDAY

FOOD
Breakfast

Lunch

Snacks

Dinner

EXERCISE
Steps

Workout

Exercise 1

Exercise 2

Exercise 3

Exercise 4

Water

Calories IN	Calories OUT	Sleep

THURSDAY

FOOD
Breakfast

Lunch

Snacks

Dinner

EXERCISE
Steps

Workout

Exercise 1

Exercise 2

Exercise 3

Exercise 4

Water

Calories IN	Calories OUT	Sleep

FRIDAY

FOOD
Breakfast

Lunch

Snacks

Dinner

EXERCISE
Steps

Workout

Exercise 1

Exercise 2

Exercise 3

Exercise 4

Water

Calories IN	Calories OUT	Sleep

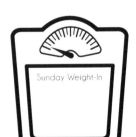

Sunday Weight-In

GOALS AND THINGS TO WORK ON THIS WEEK:

WEEK #9

TUESDAY

FOOD

Breakfast

Lunch

Snacks

Dinner

EXERCISE

Steps

Workout

Exercise 1

Exercise 2

Exercise 3

Exercise 4

Water

Calories IN	Calories OUT	Sleep

WEDNESDAY

FOOD

Breakfast

Lunch

Snacks

Dinner

EXERCISE

Steps

Workout

Exercise 1

Exercise 2

Exercise 3

Exercise 4

Water

Calories IN	Calories OUT	Sleep

SATURDAY

FOOD

Breakfast

Lunch

Snacks

Dinner

EXERCISE

Steps

Workout

Exercise 1

Exercise 2

Exercise 3

Exercise 4

Water

Calories IN	Calories OUT	Sleep

WEEKLY SUMMARY

WORKOUTS THIS WEEK

HOW HAPPY ARE YOU WITH YOUR PROGRESS

AVERAGE WATER

Calories IN	Calories OUT	Sleep

GOALS AND THINGS TO WORK ON THIS WEEK:

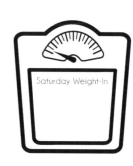

Saturday Weight-In

WEEK #10

SUNDAY

FOOD

Breakfast

Lunch

Snacks

Dinner

EXERCISE

Steps

Workout

Exercise 1

Exercise 2

Exercise 3

Exercise 4

Water

Calories IN	Calories OUT	Sleep

MONDAY

FOOD

Breakfast

Lunch

Snacks

Dinner

EXERCISE

Steps

Workout

Exercise 1

Exercise 2

Exercise 3

Exercise 4

Water

Calories IN	Calories OUT	Sleep

THURSDAY

FOOD

Breakfast

Lunch

Snacks

Dinner

EXERCISE

Steps

Workout

Exercise 1

Exercise 2

Exercise 3

Exercise 4

Water

Calories IN	Calories OUT	Sleep

FRIDAY

FOOD

Breakfast

Lunch

Snacks

Dinner

EXERCISE

Steps

Workout

Exercise 1

Exercise 2

Exercise 3

Exercise 4

Water

Calories IN	Calories OUT	Sleep

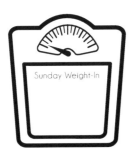

Sunday Weight-In

GOALS AND THINGS TO WORK ON THIS WEEK:

WEEK #10

TUESDAY

FOOD

Breakfast

Lunch

Snacks

Dinner

EXERCISE

Steps

Workout

Exercise 1

Exercise 2

Exercise 3

Exercise 4

Water

Calories IN	Calories OUT	Sleep

WEDNESDAY

FOOD

Breakfast

Lunch

Snacks

Dinner

EXERCISE

Steps

Workout

Exercise 1

Exercise 2

Exercise 3

Exercise 4

Water

Calories IN	Calories OUT	Sleep

SATURDAY

FOOD

Breakfast

Lunch

Snacks

Dinner

EXERCISE

Steps

Workout

Exercise 1

Exercise 2

Exercise 3

Exercise 4

Water

Calories IN	Calories OUT	Sleep

WEEKLY SUMMARY

WORKOUTS THIS WEEK

HOW HAPPY ARE YOU WITH YOUR PROGRESS

AVERAGE WATER

Calories IN	Calories OUT	Sleep

GOALS AND THINGS TO WORK ON THIS WEEK:

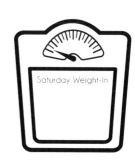

Saturday Weight-In

WEEK #11

SUNDAY

FOOD

Breakfast

Lunch

Snacks

Dinner

EXERCISE

Steps

Workout

Exercise 1

Exercise 2

Exercise 3

Exercise 4

Water

Calories IN	Calories OUT	Sleep

MONDAY

FOOD

Breakfast

Lunch

Snacks

Dinner

EXERCISE

Steps

Workout

Exercise 1

Exercise 2

Exercise 3

Exercise 4

Water

Calories IN	Calories OUT	Sleep

THURSDAY

FOOD

Breakfast

Lunch

Snacks

Dinner

EXERCISE

Steps

Workout

Exercise 1

Exercise 2

Exercise 3

Exercise 4

Water

Calories IN	Calories OUT	Sleep

FRIDAY

FOOD

Breakfast

Lunch

Snacks

Dinner

EXERCISE

Steps

Workout

Exercise 1

Exercise 2

Exercise 3

Exercise 4

Water

Calories IN	Calories OUT	Sleep

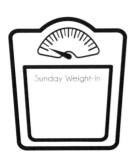

Sunday Weight-In

GOALS AND THINGS TO WORK ON THIS WEEK:

TUESDAY

FOOD

Breakfast

Lunch

Snacks

Dinner

EXERCISE

Steps

Workout

Exercise 1

Exercise 2

Exercise 3

Exercise 4

Water

Calories IN	Calories OUT	Sleep

WEDNESDAY

FOOD

Breakfast

Lunch

Snacks

Dinner

EXERCISE

Steps

Workout

Exercise 1

Exercise 2

Exercise 3

Exercise 4

Water

Calories IN	Calories OUT	Sleep

SATURDAY

FOOD

Breakfast

Lunch

Snacks

Dinner

EXERCISE

Steps

Workout

Exercise 1

Exercise 2

Exercise 3

Exercise 4

Water

Calories IN	Calories OUT	Sleep

WEEKLY SUMMARY

WORKOUTS THIS WEEK

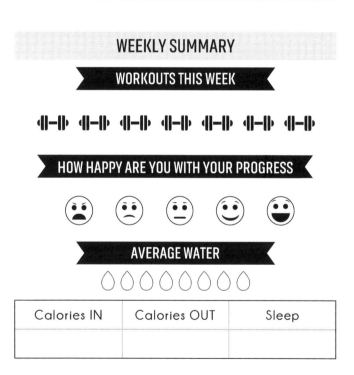

HOW HAPPY ARE YOU WITH YOUR PROGRESS

AVERAGE WATER

Calories IN	Calories OUT	Sleep

GOALS AND THINGS TO WORK ON THIS WEEK:

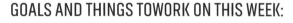

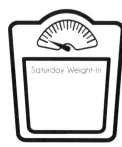

Saturday Weight-In

WEEK #12

SUNDAY

FOOD
Breakfast

Lunch

Snacks

Dinner

EXERCISE
Steps

Workout

Exercise 1

Exercise 2

Exercise 3

Exercise 4

Water

Calories IN	Calories OUT	Sleep

MONDAY

FOOD
Breakfast

Lunch

Snacks

Dinner

EXERCISE
Steps

Workout

Exercise 1

Exercise 2

Exercise 3

Exercise 4

Water

Calories IN	Calories OUT	Sleep

THURSDAY

FOOD
Breakfast

Lunch

Snacks

Dinner

EXERCISE
Steps

Workout

Exercise 1

Exercise 2

Exercise 3

Exercise 4

Water

Calories IN	Calories OUT	Sleep

FRIDAY

FOOD
Breakfast

Lunch

Snacks

Dinner

EXERCISE
Steps

Workout

Exercise 1

Exercise 2

Exercise 3

Exercise 4

Water

Calories IN	Calories OUT	Sleep

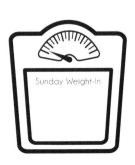

Sunday Weight-In

GOALS AND THINGS TO WORK ON THIS WEEK:

TUESDAY

FOOD

Breakfast

Lunch

Snacks

Dinner

EXERCISE

Steps

Workout

Exercise 1

Exercise 2

Exercise 3

Exercise 4

Water

Calories IN	Calories OUT	Sleep

WEDNESDAY

FOOD

Breakfast

Lunch

Snacks

Dinner

EXERCISE

Steps

Workout

Exercise 1

Exercise 2

Exercise 3

Exercise 4

Water

Calories IN	Calories OUT	Sleep

SATURDAY

FOOD

Breakfast

Lunch

Snacks

Dinner

EXERCISE

Steps

Workout

Exercise 1

Exercise 2

Exercise 3

Exercise 4

Water

Calories IN	Calories OUT	Sleep

WEEKLY SUMMARY

WORKOUTS THIS WEEK

HOW HAPPY ARE YOU WITH YOUR PROGRESS

AVERAGE WATER

Calories IN	Calories OUT	Sleep

GOALS AND THINGS TOWORK ON THIS WEEK:

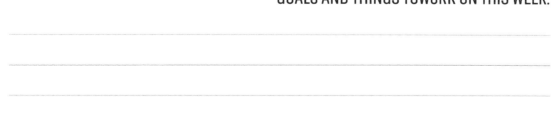

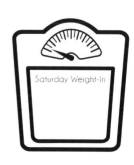

Saturday Weight-In

WEEK #13

SUNDAY

FOOD

Breakfast

Lunch

Snacks

Dinner

EXERCISE

Steps

Workout

Exercise 1

Exercise 2

Exercise 3

Exercise 4

Water

Calories IN	Calories OUT	Sleep

MONDAY

FOOD

Breakfast

Lunch

Snacks

Dinner

EXERCISE

Steps

Workout

Exercise 1

Exercise 2

Exercise 3

Exercise 4

Water

Calories IN	Calories OUT	Sleep

THURSDAY

FOOD

Breakfast

Lunch

Snacks

Dinner

EXERCISE

Steps

Workout

Exercise 1

Exercise 2

Exercise 3

Exercise 4

Water

Calories IN	Calories OUT	Sleep

FRIDAY

FOOD

Breakfast

Lunch

Snacks

Dinner

EXERCISE

Steps

Workout

Exercise 1

Exercise 2

Exercise 3

Exercise 4

Water

Calories IN	Calories OUT	Sleep

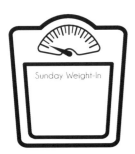

Sunday Weight-In

GOALS AND THINGS TO WORK ON THIS WEEK:

TUESDAY

FOOD

Breakfast

Lunch

Snacks

Dinner

EXERCISE

Steps

Workout

Exercise 1

Exercise 2

Exercise 3

Exercise 4

Water

Calories IN	Calories OUT	Sleep

WEDNESDAY

FOOD

Breakfast

Lunch

Snacks

Dinner

EXERCISE

Steps

Workout

Exercise 1

Exercise 2

Exercise 3

Exercise 4

Water

Calories IN	Calories OUT	Sleep

SATURDAY

FOOD

Breakfast

Lunch

Snacks

Dinner

EXERCISE

Steps

Workout

Exercise 1

Exercise 2

Exercise 3

Exercise 4

Water

Calories IN	Calories OUT	Sleep

WEEKLY SUMMARY

WORKOUTS THIS WEEK

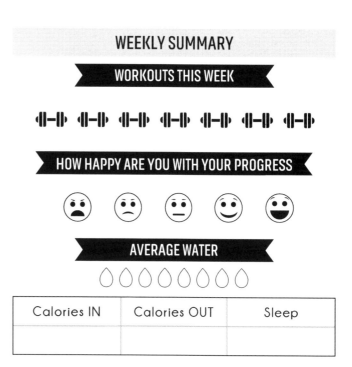

HOW HAPPY ARE YOU WITH YOUR PROGRESS

AVERAGE WATER

Calories IN	Calories OUT	Sleep

GOALS AND THINGS TO WORK ON THIS WEEK:

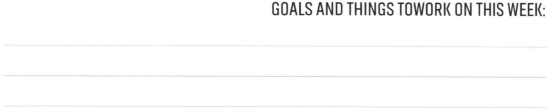
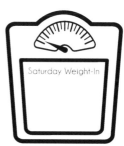

Saturday Weight-In

WEEK #14

SUNDAY

FOOD

Breakfast

Lunch

Snacks

Dinner

EXERCISE

Steps

Workout

Exercise 1

Exercise 2

Exercise 3

Exercise 4

Water

Calories IN	Calories OUT	Sleep

MONDAY

FOOD

Breakfast

Lunch

Snacks

Dinner

EXERCISE

Steps

Workout

Exercise 1

Exercise 2

Exercise 3

Exercise 4

Water

Calories IN	Calories OUT	Sleep

THURSDAY

FOOD

Breakfast

Lunch

Snacks

Dinner

EXERCISE

Steps

Workout

Exercise 1

Exercise 2

Exercise 3

Exercise 4

Water

Calories IN	Calories OUT	Sleep

FRIDAY

FOOD

Breakfast

Lunch

Snacks

Dinner

EXERCISE

Steps

Workout

Exercise 1

Exercise 2

Exercise 3

Exercise 4

Water

Calories IN	Calories OUT	Sleep

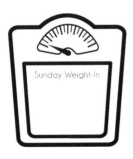

Sunday Weight-In

GOALS AND THINGS TOWORK ON THIS WEEK:

TUESDAY

FOOD

Breakfast

Lunch

Snacks

Dinner

EXERCISE

Steps

Workout

Exercise 1

Exercise 2

Exercise 3

Exercise 4

Water

Calories IN	Calories OUT	Sleep

WEDNESDAY

FOOD

Breakfast

Lunch

Snacks

Dinner

EXERCISE

Steps

Workout

Exercise 1

Exercise 2

Exercise 3

Exercise 4

Water

Calories IN	Calories OUT	Sleep

SATURDAY

FOOD

Breakfast

Lunch

Snacks

Dinner

EXERCISE

Steps

Workout

Exercise 1

Exercise 2

Exercise 3

Exercise 4

Water

Calories IN	Calories OUT	Sleep

WEEKLY SUMMARY

WORKOUTS THIS WEEK

HOW HAPPY ARE YOU WITH YOUR PROGRESS

AVERAGE WATER

Calories IN	Calories OUT	Sleep

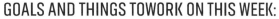

GOALS AND THINGS TOWORK ON THIS WEEK:

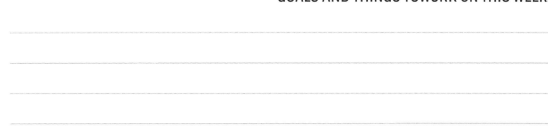

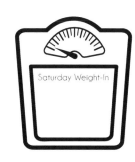

Saturday Weight-In

WEEK #15

SUNDAY

FOOD
Breakfast

Lunch

Snacks

Dinner

EXERCISE
Steps

Workout

Exercise 1

Exercise 2

Exercise 3

Exercise 4

Water

Calories IN	Calories OUT	Sleep

MONDAY

FOOD
Breakfast

Lunch

Snacks

Dinner

EXERCISE
Steps

Workout

Exercise 1

Exercise 2

Exercise 3

Exercise 4

Water

Calories IN	Calories OUT	Sleep

THURSDAY

FOOD
Breakfast

Lunch

Snacks

Dinner

EXERCISE
Steps

Workout

Exercise 1

Exercise 2

Exercise 3

Exercise 4

Water

Calories IN	Calories OUT	Sleep

FRIDAY

FOOD
Breakfast

Lunch

Snacks

Dinner

EXERCISE
Steps

Workout

Exercise 1

Exercise 2

Exercise 3

Exercise 4

Water

Calories IN	Calories OUT	Sleep

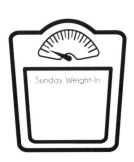

Sunday Weight-In

GOALS AND THINGS TO WORK ON THIS WEEK:

TUESDAY

FOOD

Breakfast

Lunch

Snacks

Dinner

EXERCISE

Steps

Workout

Exercise 1

Exercise 2

Exercise 3

Exercise 4

Water

Calories IN	Calories OUT	Sleep

WEDNESDAY

FOOD

Breakfast

Lunch

Snacks

Dinner

EXERCISE

Steps

Workout

Exercise 1

Exercise 2

Exercise 3

Exercise 4

Water

Calories IN	Calories OUT	Sleep

SATURDAY

FOOD

Breakfast

Lunch

Snacks

Dinner

EXERCISE

Steps

Workout

Exercise 1

Exercise 2

Exercise 3

Exercise 4

Water

Calories IN	Calories OUT	Sleep

WEEKLY SUMMARY

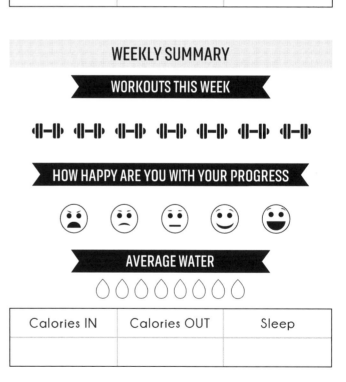

WORKOUTS THIS WEEK

HOW HAPPY ARE YOU WITH YOUR PROGRESS

AVERAGE WATER

Calories IN	Calories OUT	Sleep

GOALS AND THINGS TO WORK ON THIS WEEK:

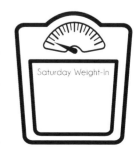

Saturday Weight-In

WEEK #16

SUNDAY

FOOD	EXERCISE
Breakfast	Steps
	Workout
Lunch	Exercise 1
	Exercise 2
Snacks	Exercise 3
	Exercise 4
Dinner	Water

Calories IN	Calories OUT	Sleep

MONDAY

FOOD	EXERCISE
Breakfast	Steps
	Workout
Lunch	Exercise 1
	Exercise 2
Snacks	Exercise 3
	Exercise 4
Dinner	Water

Calories IN	Calories OUT	Sleep

THURSDAY

FOOD	EXERCISE
Breakfast	Steps
	Workout
Lunch	Exercise 1
	Exercise 2
Snacks	Exercise 3
	Exercise 4
Dinner	Water

Calories IN	Calories OUT	Sleep

FRIDAY

FOOD	EXERCISE
Breakfast	Steps
	Workout
Lunch	Exercise 1
	Exercise 2
Snacks	Exercise 3
	Exercise 4
Dinner	Water

Calories IN	Calories OUT	Sleep

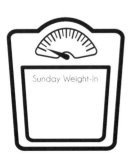

Sunday Weight-In

GOALS AND THINGS TO WORK ON THIS WEEK:

TUESDAY

FOOD

Breakfast

Lunch

Snacks

Dinner

EXERCISE

Steps

Workout

Exercise 1

Exercise 2

Exercise 3

Exercise 4

Water

Calories IN	Calories OUT	Sleep

WEDNESDAY

FOOD

Breakfast

Lunch

Snacks

Dinner

EXERCISE

Steps

Workout

Exercise 1

Exercise 2

Exercise 3

Exercise 4

Water

Calories IN	Calories OUT	Sleep

SATURDAY

FOOD

Breakfast

Lunch

Snacks

Dinner

EXERCISE

Steps

Workout

Exercise 1

Exercise 2

Exercise 3

Exercise 4

Water

Calories IN	Calories OUT	Sleep

WEEKLY SUMMARY

WORKOUTS THIS WEEK

HOW HAPPY ARE YOU WITH YOUR PROGRESS

AVERAGE WATER

Calories IN	Calories OUT	Sleep

GOALS AND THINGS TOWORK ON THIS WEEK:

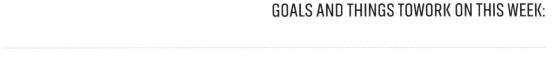

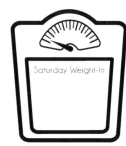

Saturday Weight-In

WEEK #17

SUNDAY

FOOD
Breakfast

Lunch

Snacks

Dinner

EXERCISE
Steps

Workout

Exercise 1

Exercise 2

Exercise 3

Exercise 4

Water

Calories IN	Calories OUT	Sleep

MONDAY

FOOD
Breakfast

Lunch

Snacks

Dinner

EXERCISE
Steps

Workout

Exercise 1

Exercise 2

Exercise 3

Exercise 4

Water

Calories IN	Calories OUT	Sleep

THURSDAY

FOOD
Breakfast

Lunch

Snacks

Dinner

EXERCISE
Steps

Workout

Exercise 1

Exercise 2

Exercise 3

Exercise 4

Water

Calories IN	Calories OUT	Sleep

FRIDAY

FOOD
Breakfast

Lunch

Snacks

Dinner

EXERCISE
Steps

Workout

Exercise 1

Exercise 2

Exercise 3

Exercise 4

Water

Calories IN	Calories OUT	Sleep

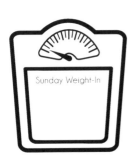

Sunday Weight-In

GOALS AND THINGS TO WORK ON THIS WEEK:

TUESDAY

FOOD

Breakfast

Lunch

Snacks

Dinner

EXERCISE

Steps

Workout

Exercise 1

Exercise 2

Exercise 3

Exercise 4

Water

Calories IN	Calories OUT	Sleep

WEDNESDAY

FOOD

Breakfast

Lunch

Snacks

Dinner

EXERCISE

Steps

Workout

Exercise 1

Exercise 2

Exercise 3

Exercise 4

Water

Calories IN	Calories OUT	Sleep

SATURDAY

FOOD

Breakfast

Lunch

Snacks

Dinner

EXERCISE

Steps

Workout

Exercise 1

Exercise 2

Exercise 3

Exercise 4

Water

Calories IN	Calories OUT	Sleep

WEEKLY SUMMARY

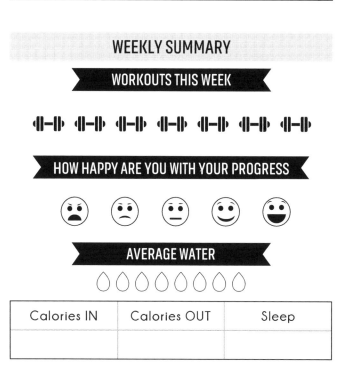

WORKOUTS THIS WEEK

HOW HAPPY ARE YOU WITH YOUR PROGRESS

AVERAGE WATER

Calories IN	Calories OUT	Sleep

GOALS AND THINGS TO WORK ON THIS WEEK:

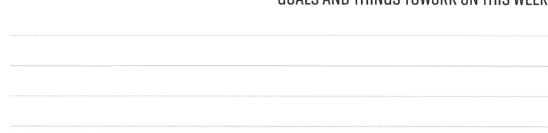

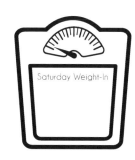

Saturday Weight-In

WEEK #18

SUNDAY

FOOD

Breakfast

Lunch

Snacks

Dinner

EXERCISE

Steps

Workout

Exercise 1

Exercise 2

Exercise 3

Exercise 4

Water

Calories IN	Calories OUT	Sleep

MONDAY

FOOD

Breakfast

Lunch

Snacks

Dinner

EXERCISE

Steps

Workout

Exercise 1

Exercise 2

Exercise 3

Exercise 4

Water

Calories IN	Calories OUT	Sleep

THURSDAY

FOOD

Breakfast

Lunch

Snacks

Dinner

EXERCISE

Steps

Workout

Exercise 1

Exercise 2

Exercise 3

Exercise 4

Water

Calories IN	Calories OUT	Sleep

FRIDAY

FOOD

Breakfast

Lunch

Snacks

Dinner

EXERCISE

Steps

Workout

Exercise 1

Exercise 2

Exercise 3

Exercise 4

Water

Calories IN	Calories OUT	Sleep

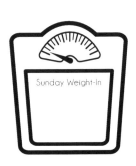

Sunday Weight-In

GOALS AND THINGS TO WORK ON THIS WEEK:

TUESDAY

FOOD	EXERCISE
Breakfast	Steps
	Workout
Lunch	Exercise 1
	Exercise 2
Snacks	Exercise 3
	Exercise 4
Dinner	Water

Calories IN	Calories OUT	Sleep

WEDNESDAY

FOOD	EXERCISE
Breakfast	Steps
	Workout
Lunch	Exercise 1
	Exercise 2
Snacks	Exercise 3
	Exercise 4
Dinner	Water

Calories IN	Calories OUT	Sleep

SATURDAY

FOOD	EXERCISE
Breakfast	Steps
	Workout
Lunch	Exercise 1
	Exercise 2
Snacks	Exercise 3
	Exercise 4
Dinner	Water

Calories IN	Calories OUT	Sleep

WEEKLY SUMMARY

WORKOUTS THIS WEEK

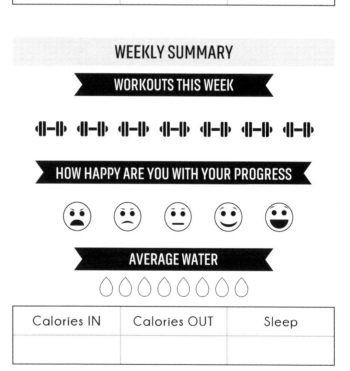

HOW HAPPY ARE YOU WITH YOUR PROGRESS

AVERAGE WATER

Calories IN	Calories OUT	Sleep

GOALS AND THINGS TO WORK ON THIS WEEK:

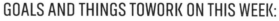
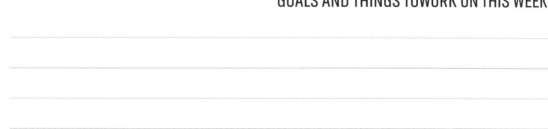
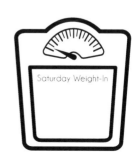

Saturday Weight-In

WEEK #19

SUNDAY

FOOD

Breakfast

Lunch

Snacks

Dinner

EXERCISE

Steps

Workout

Exercise 1

Exercise 2

Exercise 3

Exercise 4

Water

Calories IN	Calories OUT	Sleep

MONDAY

FOOD

Breakfast

Lunch

Snacks

Dinner

EXERCISE

Steps

Workout

Exercise 1

Exercise 2

Exercise 3

Exercise 4

Water

Calories IN	Calories OUT	Sleep

THURSDAY

FOOD

Breakfast

Lunch

Snacks

Dinner

EXERCISE

Steps

Workout

Exercise 1

Exercise 2

Exercise 3

Exercise 4

Water

Calories IN	Calories OUT	Sleep

FRIDAY

FOOD

Breakfast

Lunch

Snacks

Dinner

EXERCISE

Steps

Workout

Exercise 1

Exercise 2

Exercise 3

Exercise 4

Water

Calories IN	Calories OUT	Sleep

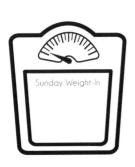

Sunday Weight-In

GOALS AND THINGS TO WORK ON THIS WEEK:

TUESDAY

FOOD

Breakfast

Lunch

Snacks

Dinner

EXERCISE

Steps

Workout

Exercise 1

Exercise 2

Exercise 3

Exercise 4

Water

Calories IN	Calories OUT	Sleep

WEDNESDAY

FOOD

Breakfast

Lunch

Snacks

Dinner

EXERCISE

Steps

Workout

Exercise 1

Exercise 2

Exercise 3

Exercise 4

Water

Calories IN	Calories OUT	Sleep

SATURDAY

FOOD

Breakfast

Lunch

Snacks

Dinner

EXERCISE

Steps

Workout

Exercise 1

Exercise 2

Exercise 3

Exercise 4

Water

Calories IN	Calories OUT	Sleep

WEEKLY SUMMARY

WORKOUTS THIS WEEK

HOW HAPPY ARE YOU WITH YOUR PROGRESS

AVERAGE WATER

Calories IN	Calories OUT	Sleep

GOALS AND THINGS TOWORK ON THIS WEEK:

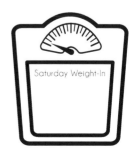

Saturday Weight-In

WEEK #20

SUNDAY

FOOD
Breakfast

Lunch

Snacks

Dinner

EXERCISE
Steps

Workout

Exercise 1

Exercise 2

Exercise 3

Exercise 4

Water

Calories IN	Calories OUT	Sleep

MONDAY

FOOD
Breakfast

Lunch

Snacks

Dinner

EXERCISE
Steps

Workout

Exercise 1

Exercise 2

Exercise 3

Exercise 4

Water

Calories IN	Calories OUT	Sleep

THURSDAY

FOOD
Breakfast

Lunch

Snacks

Dinner

EXERCISE
Steps

Workout

Exercise 1

Exercise 2

Exercise 3

Exercise 4

Water

Calories IN	Calories OUT	Sleep

FRIDAY

FOOD
Breakfast

Lunch

Snacks

Dinner

EXERCISE
Steps

Workout

Exercise 1

Exercise 2

Exercise 3

Exercise 4

Water

Calories IN	Calories OUT	Sleep

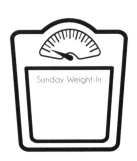

Sunday Weight-In

GOALS AND THINGS TO WORK ON THIS WEEK:

TUESDAY

FOOD

Breakfast

Lunch

Snacks

Dinner

EXERCISE

Steps

Workout

Exercise 1

Exercise 2

Exercise 3

Exercise 4

Water

Calories IN	Calories OUT	Sleep

WEDNESDAY

FOOD

Breakfast

Lunch

Snacks

Dinner

EXERCISE

Steps

Workout

Exercise 1

Exercise 2

Exercise 3

Exercise 4

Water

Calories IN	Calories OUT	Sleep

SATURDAY

FOOD

Breakfast

Lunch

Snacks

Dinner

EXERCISE

Steps

Workout

Exercise 1

Exercise 2

Exercise 3

Exercise 4

Water

Calories IN	Calories OUT	Sleep

WEEKLY SUMMARY

WORKOUTS THIS WEEK

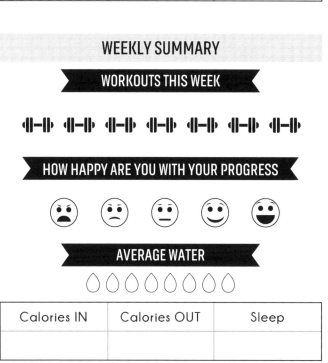

HOW HAPPY ARE YOU WITH YOUR PROGRESS

AVERAGE WATER

Calories IN	Calories OUT	Sleep

GOALS AND THINGS TO WORK ON THIS WEEK:

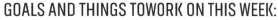

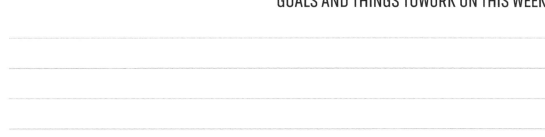

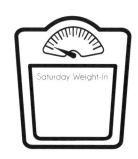

Saturday Weight-In

WEEK #21

SUNDAY

FOOD	EXERCISE
Breakfast	Steps
	Workout
Lunch	Exercise 1
	Exercise 2
Snacks	Exercise 3
	Exercise 4
Dinner	Water

Calories IN	Calories OUT	Sleep

MONDAY

FOOD	EXERCISE
Breakfast	Steps
	Workout
Lunch	Exercise 1
	Exercise 2
Snacks	Exercise 3
	Exercise 4
Dinner	Water

Calories IN	Calories OUT	Sleep

THURSDAY

FOOD	EXERCISE
Breakfast	Steps
	Workout
Lunch	Exercise 1
	Exercise 2
Snacks	Exercise 3
	Exercise 4
Dinner	Water

Calories IN	Calories OUT	Sleep

FRIDAY

FOOD	EXERCISE
Breakfast	Steps
	Workout
Lunch	Exercise 1
	Exercise 2
Snacks	Exercise 3
	Exercise 4
Dinner	Water

Calories IN	Calories OUT	Sleep

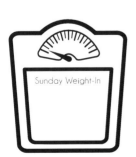

Sunday Weight-In

GOALS AND THINGS TO WORK ON THIS WEEK:

TUESDAY

FOOD

Breakfast

Lunch

Snacks

Dinner

EXERCISE

Steps

Workout

Exercise 1

Exercise 2

Exercise 3

Exercise 4

Water

Calories IN	Calories OUT	Sleep

WEDNESDAY

FOOD

Breakfast

Lunch

Snacks

Dinner

EXERCISE

Steps

Workout

Exercise 1

Exercise 2

Exercise 3

Exercise 4

Water

Calories IN	Calories OUT	Sleep

SATURDAY

FOOD

Breakfast

Lunch

Snacks

Dinner

EXERCISE

Steps

Workout

Exercise 1

Exercise 2

Exercise 3

Exercise 4

Water

Calories IN	Calories OUT	Sleep

WEEKLY SUMMARY

WORKOUTS THIS WEEK

HOW HAPPY ARE YOU WITH YOUR PROGRESS

AVERAGE WATER

Calories IN	Calories OUT	Sleep

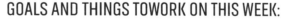

GOALS AND THINGS TO WORK ON THIS WEEK:

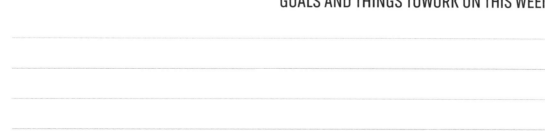

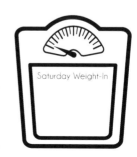

Saturday Weight-In

WEEK #22

SUNDAY

FOOD

Breakfast

Lunch

Snacks

Dinner

EXERCISE

Steps

Workout

Exercise 1

Exercise 2

Exercise 3

Exercise 4

Water

Calories IN	Calories OUT	Sleep

MONDAY

FOOD

Breakfast

Lunch

Snacks

Dinner

EXERCISE

Steps

Workout

Exercise 1

Exercise 2

Exercise 3

Exercise 4

Water

Calories IN	Calories OUT	Sleep

THURSDAY

FOOD

Breakfast

Lunch

Snacks

Dinner

EXERCISE

Steps

Workout

Exercise 1

Exercise 2

Exercise 3

Exercise 4

Water

Calories IN	Calories OUT	Sleep

FRIDAY

FOOD

Breakfast

Lunch

Snacks

Dinner

EXERCISE

Steps

Workout

Exercise 1

Exercise 2

Exercise 3

Exercise 4

Water

Calories IN	Calories OUT	Sleep

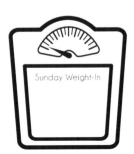

Sunday Weight-In

GOALS AND THINGS TOWORK ON THIS WEEK:

TUESDAY

FOOD

Breakfast

Lunch

Snacks

Dinner

EXERCISE

Steps

Workout

Exercise 1

Exercise 2

Exercise 3

Exercise 4

Water

Calories IN	Calories OUT	Sleep

WEDNESDAY

FOOD

Breakfast

Lunch

Snacks

Dinner

EXERCISE

Steps

Workout

Exercise 1

Exercise 2

Exercise 3

Exercise 4

Water

Calories IN	Calories OUT	Sleep

SATURDAY

FOOD

Breakfast

Lunch

Snacks

Dinner

EXERCISE

Steps

Workout

Exercise 1

Exercise 2

Exercise 3

Exercise 4

Water

Calories IN	Calories OUT	Sleep

WEEKLY SUMMARY

WORKOUTS THIS WEEK

HOW HAPPY ARE YOU WITH YOUR PROGRESS

AVERAGE WATER

Calories IN	Calories OUT	Sleep

GOALS AND THINGS TO WORK ON THIS WEEK:

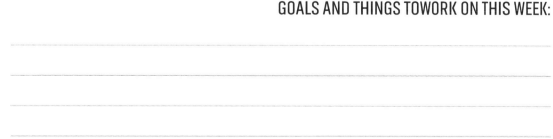

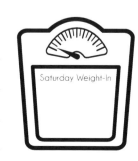

Saturday Weight-In

WEEK #23

SUNDAY

FOOD
Breakfast

Lunch

Snacks

Dinner

EXERCISE
Steps

Workout

Exercise 1

Exercise 2

Exercise 3

Exercise 4

Water

Calories IN	Calories OUT	Sleep

MONDAY

FOOD
Breakfast

Lunch

Snacks

Dinner

EXERCISE
Steps

Workout

Exercise 1

Exercise 2

Exercise 3

Exercise 4

Water

Calories IN	Calories OUT	Sleep

THURSDAY

FOOD
Breakfast

Lunch

Snacks

Dinner

EXERCISE
Steps

Workout

Exercise 1

Exercise 2

Exercise 3

Exercise 4

Water

Calories IN	Calories OUT	Sleep

FRIDAY

FOOD
Breakfast

Lunch

Snacks

Dinner

EXERCISE
Steps

Workout

Exercise 1

Exercise 2

Exercise 3

Exercise 4

Water

Calories IN	Calories OUT	Sleep

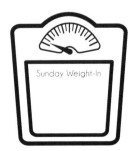

Sunday Weight-In

GOALS AND THINGS TO WORK ON THIS WEEK:

TUESDAY

FOOD

Breakfast

Lunch

Snacks

Dinner

EXERCISE

Steps

Workout

Exercise 1

Exercise 2

Exercise 3

Exercise 4

Water

Calories IN	Calories OUT	Sleep

WEDNESDAY

FOOD

Breakfast

Lunch

Snacks

Dinner

EXERCISE

Steps

Workout

Exercise 1

Exercise 2

Exercise 3

Exercise 4

Water

Calories IN	Calories OUT	Sleep

SATURDAY

FOOD

Breakfast

Lunch

Snacks

Dinner

EXERCISE

Steps

Workout

Exercise 1

Exercise 2

Exercise 3

Exercise 4

Water

Calories IN	Calories OUT	Sleep

WEEKLY SUMMARY

WORKOUTS THIS WEEK

HOW HAPPY ARE YOU WITH YOUR PROGRESS

AVERAGE WATER

Calories IN	Calories OUT	Sleep

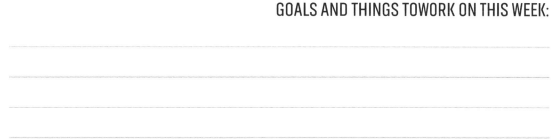

GOALS AND THINGS TOWORK ON THIS WEEK:

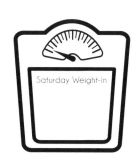

Saturday Weight-In

WEEK #24

SUNDAY

FOOD

Breakfast

Lunch

Snacks

Dinner

EXERCISE

Steps

Workout

Exercise 1

Exercise 2

Exercise 3

Exercise 4

Water

Calories IN	Calories OUT	Sleep

MONDAY

FOOD

Breakfast

Lunch

Snacks

Dinner

EXERCISE

Steps

Workout

Exercise 1

Exercise 2

Exercise 3

Exercise 4

Water

Calories IN	Calories OUT	Sleep

THURSDAY

FOOD

Breakfast

Lunch

Snacks

Dinner

EXERCISE

Steps

Workout

Exercise 1

Exercise 2

Exercise 3

Exercise 4

Water

Calories IN	Calories OUT	Sleep

FRIDAY

FOOD

Breakfast

Lunch

Snacks

Dinner

EXERCISE

Steps

Workout

Exercise 1

Exercise 2

Exercise 3

Exercise 4

Water

Calories IN	Calories OUT	Sleep

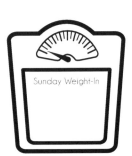

Sunday Weight-In

GOALS AND THINGS TO WORK ON THIS WEEK:

TUESDAY

FOOD

Breakfast

Lunch

Snacks

Dinner

EXERCISE

Steps

Workout

Exercise 1

Exercise 2

Exercise 3

Exercise 4

Water

Calories IN	Calories OUT	Sleep

WEDNESDAY

FOOD

Breakfast

Lunch

Snacks

Dinner

EXERCISE

Steps

Workout

Exercise 1

Exercise 2

Exercise 3

Exercise 4

Water

Calories IN	Calories OUT	Sleep

SATURDAY

FOOD

Breakfast

Lunch

Snacks

Dinner

EXERCISE

Steps

Workout

Exercise 1

Exercise 2

Exercise 3

Exercise 4

Water

Calories IN	Calories OUT	Sleep

WEEKLY SUMMARY

WORKOUTS THIS WEEK

HOW HAPPY ARE YOU WITH YOUR PROGRESS

AVERAGE WATER

Calories IN	Calories OUT	Sleep

GOALS AND THINGS TO WORK ON THIS WEEK:

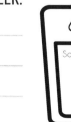

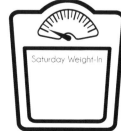

Saturday Weight-In

WEEK #25

SUNDAY

FOOD

Breakfast

Lunch

Snacks

Dinner

EXERCISE

Steps

Workout

Exercise 1

Exercise 2

Exercise 3

Exercise 4

Water

Calories IN	Calories OUT	Sleep

MONDAY

FOOD

Breakfast

Lunch

Snacks

Dinner

EXERCISE

Steps

Workout

Exercise 1

Exercise 2

Exercise 3

Exercise 4

Water

Calories IN	Calories OUT	Sleep

THURSDAY

FOOD

Breakfast

Lunch

Snacks

Dinner

EXERCISE

Steps

Workout

Exercise 1

Exercise 2

Exercise 3

Exercise 4

Water

Calories IN	Calories OUT	Sleep

FRIDAY

FOOD

Breakfast

Lunch

Snacks

Dinner

EXERCISE

Steps

Workout

Exercise 1

Exercise 2

Exercise 3

Exercise 4

Water

Calories IN	Calories OUT	Sleep

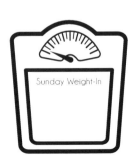

Sunday Weight-In

GOALS AND THINGS TO WORK ON THIS WEEK:

TUESDAY

FOOD

Breakfast

Lunch

Snacks

Dinner

EXERCISE

Steps

Workout

Exercise 1

Exercise 2

Exercise 3

Exercise 4

Water

Calories IN	Calories OUT	Sleep

WEDNESDAY

FOOD

Breakfast

Lunch

Snacks

Dinner

EXERCISE

Steps

Workout

Exercise 1

Exercise 2

Exercise 3

Exercise 4

Water

Calories IN	Calories OUT	Sleep

SATURDAY

FOOD

Breakfast

Lunch

Snacks

Dinner

EXERCISE

Steps

Workout

Exercise 1

Exercise 2

Exercise 3

Exercise 4

Water

Calories IN	Calories OUT	Sleep

WEEKLY SUMMARY

WORKOUTS THIS WEEK

HOW HAPPY ARE YOU WITH YOUR PROGRESS

AVERAGE WATER

Calories IN	Calories OUT	Sleep

GOALS AND THINGS TO WORK ON THIS WEEK:

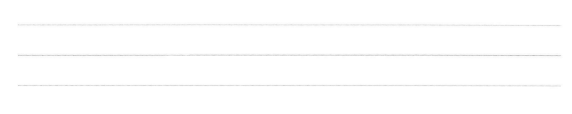

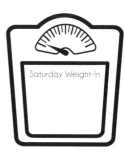

Saturday Weight-In

WEEK #26

SUNDAY

FOOD
Breakfast

Lunch

Snacks

Dinner

EXERCISE
Steps

Workout

Exercise 1

Exercise 2

Exercise 3

Exercise 4

Water
🝙🝙🝙🝙🝙🝙🝙🝙

Calories IN	Calories OUT	Sleep

MONDAY

FOOD
Breakfast

Lunch

Snacks

Dinner

EXERCISE
Steps

Workout

Exercise 1

Exercise 2

Exercise 3

Exercise 4

Water
🝙🝙🝙🝙🝙🝙🝙🝙

Calories IN	Calories OUT	Sleep

THURSDAY

FOOD
Breakfast

Lunch

Snacks

Dinner

EXERCISE
Steps

Workout

Exercise 1

Exercise 2

Exercise 3

Exercise 4

Water
🝙🝙🝙🝙🝙🝙🝙🝙

Calories IN	Calories OUT	Sleep

FRIDAY

FOOD
Breakfast

Lunch

Snacks

Dinner

EXERCISE
Steps

Workout

Exercise 1

Exercise 2

Exercise 3

Exercise 4

Water
🝙🝙🝙🝙🝙🝙🝙🝙

Calories IN	Calories OUT	Sleep

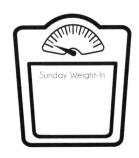

Sunday Weight-In

GOALS AND THINGS TO WORK ON THIS WEEK:

TUESDAY

FOOD

Breakfast

Lunch

Snacks

Dinner

EXERCISE

Steps

Workout

Exercise 1

Exercise 2

Exercise 3

Exercise 4

Water

Calories IN	Calories OUT	Sleep

WEDNESDAY

FOOD

Breakfast

Lunch

Snacks

Dinner

EXERCISE

Steps

Workout

Exercise 1

Exercise 2

Exercise 3

Exercise 4

Water

Calories IN	Calories OUT	Sleep

SATURDAY

FOOD

Breakfast

Lunch

Snacks

Dinner

EXERCISE

Steps

Workout

Exercise 1

Exercise 2

Exercise 3

Exercise 4

Water

Calories IN	Calories OUT	Sleep

WEEKLY SUMMARY

WORKOUTS THIS WEEK

HOW HAPPY ARE YOU WITH YOUR PROGRESS

AVERAGE WATER

Calories IN	Calories OUT	Sleep

GOALS AND THINGS TOWORK ON THIS WEEK:

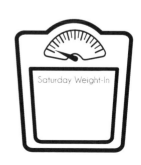

Saturday Weight-In

WEEK #27

SUNDAY

FOOD
Breakfast

Lunch

Snacks

Dinner

EXERCISE
Steps

Workout

Exercise 1

Exercise 2

Exercise 3

Exercise 4

Water

Calories IN	Calories OUT	Sleep

MONDAY

FOOD
Breakfast

Lunch

Snacks

Dinner

EXERCISE
Steps

Workout

Exercise 1

Exercise 2

Exercise 3

Exercise 4

Water

Calories IN	Calories OUT	Sleep

THURSDAY

FOOD
Breakfast

Lunch

Snacks

Dinner

EXERCISE
Steps

Workout

Exercise 1

Exercise 2

Exercise 3

Exercise 4

Water

Calories IN	Calories OUT	Sleep

FRIDAY

FOOD
Breakfast

Lunch

Snacks

Dinner

EXERCISE
Steps

Workout

Exercise 1

Exercise 2

Exercise 3

Exercise 4

Water

Calories IN	Calories OUT	Sleep

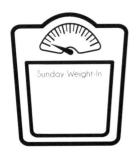

Sunday Weight-In

GOALS AND THINGS TO WORK ON THIS WEEK:

TUESDAY

FOOD

Breakfast

Lunch

Snacks

Dinner

EXERCISE

Steps

Workout

Exercise 1

Exercise 2

Exercise 3

Exercise 4

Water

Calories IN	Calories OUT	Sleep

WEDNESDAY

FOOD

Breakfast

Lunch

Snacks

Dinner

EXERCISE

Steps

Workout

Exercise 1

Exercise 2

Exercise 3

Exercise 4

Water

Calories IN	Calories OUT	Sleep

SATURDAY

FOOD

Breakfast

Lunch

Snacks

Dinner

EXERCISE

Steps

Workout

Exercise 1

Exercise 2

Exercise 3

Exercise 4

Water

Calories IN	Calories OUT	Sleep

WEEKLY SUMMARY

WORKOUTS THIS WEEK

HOW HAPPY ARE YOU WITH YOUR PROGRESS

AVERAGE WATER

Calories IN	Calories OUT	Sleep

GOALS AND THINGS TO WORK ON THIS WEEK:

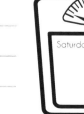

Saturday Weight-In

WEEK #28

SUNDAY

FOOD
Breakfast

Lunch

Snacks

Dinner

EXERCISE
Steps

Workout

Exercise 1

Exercise 2

Exercise 3

Exercise 4

Water

Calories IN	Calories OUT	Sleep

MONDAY

FOOD
Breakfast

Lunch

Snacks

Dinner

EXERCISE
Steps

Workout

Exercise 1

Exercise 2

Exercise 3

Exercise 4

Water

Calories IN	Calories OUT	Sleep

THURSDAY

FOOD
Breakfast

Lunch

Snacks

Dinner

EXERCISE
Steps

Workout

Exercise 1

Exercise 2

Exercise 3

Exercise 4

Water

Calories IN	Calories OUT	Sleep

FRIDAY

FOOD
Breakfast

Lunch

Snacks

Dinner

EXERCISE
Steps

Workout

Exercise 1

Exercise 2

Exercise 3

Exercise 4

Water

Calories IN	Calories OUT	Sleep

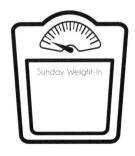

Sunday Weight-In

GOALS AND THINGS TO WORK ON THIS WEEK:

TUESDAY

FOOD

Breakfast

Lunch

Snacks

Dinner

EXERCISE

Steps

Workout

Exercise 1

Exercise 2

Exercise 3

Exercise 4

Water

Calories IN	Calories OUT	Sleep

WEDNESDAY

FOOD

Breakfast

Lunch

Snacks

Dinner

EXERCISE

Steps

Workout

Exercise 1

Exercise 2

Exercise 3

Exercise 4

Water

Calories IN	Calories OUT	Sleep

SATURDAY

FOOD

Breakfast

Lunch

Snacks

Dinner

EXERCISE

Steps

Workout

Exercise 1

Exercise 2

Exercise 3

Exercise 4

Water

Calories IN	Calories OUT	Sleep

WEEKLY SUMMARY

WORKOUTS THIS WEEK

HOW HAPPY ARE YOU WITH YOUR PROGRESS

AVERAGE WATER

Calories IN	Calories OUT	Sleep

GOALS AND THINGS TO WORK ON THIS WEEK:

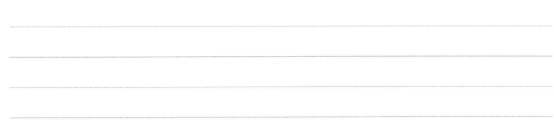

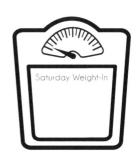

Saturday Weight-In

WEEK #29

SUNDAY

FOOD
Breakfast

Lunch

Snacks

Dinner

EXERCISE
Steps

Workout

Exercise 1

Exercise 2

Exercise 3

Exercise 4

Water

Calories IN	Calories OUT	Sleep

MONDAY

FOOD
Breakfast

Lunch

Snacks

Dinner

EXERCISE
Steps

Workout

Exercise 1

Exercise 2

Exercise 3

Exercise 4

Water

Calories IN	Calories OUT	Sleep

THURSDAY

FOOD
Breakfast

Lunch

Snacks

Dinner

EXERCISE
Steps

Workout

Exercise 1

Exercise 2

Exercise 3

Exercise 4

Water

Calories IN	Calories OUT	Sleep

FRIDAY

FOOD
Breakfast

Lunch

Snacks

Dinner

EXERCISE
Steps

Workout

Exercise 1

Exercise 2

Exercise 3

Exercise 4

Water

Calories IN	Calories OUT	Sleep

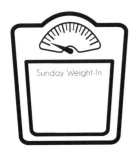

Sunday Weight-In

GOALS AND THINGS TO WORK ON THIS WEEK:

TUESDAY

FOOD

Breakfast

Lunch

Snacks

Dinner

EXERCISE

Steps

Workout

Exercise 1

Exercise 2

Exercise 3

Exercise 4

Water

Calories IN	Calories OUT	Sleep

WEDNESDAY

FOOD

Breakfast

Lunch

Snacks

Dinner

EXERCISE

Steps

Workout

Exercise 1

Exercise 2

Exercise 3

Exercise 4

Water

Calories IN	Calories OUT	Sleep

SATURDAY

FOOD

Breakfast

Lunch

Snacks

Dinner

EXERCISE

Steps

Workout

Exercise 1

Exercise 2

Exercise 3

Exercise 4

Water

Calories IN	Calories OUT	Sleep

WEEKLY SUMMARY

WORKOUTS THIS WEEK

HOW HAPPY ARE YOU WITH YOUR PROGRESS

AVERAGE WATER

Calories IN	Calories OUT	Sleep

GOALS AND THINGS TO WORK ON THIS WEEK:

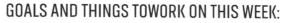

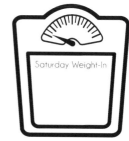

Saturday Weight-In

WEEK #30

SUNDAY

FOOD
Breakfast

Lunch

Snacks

Dinner

EXERCISE
Steps

Workout

Exercise 1

Exercise 2

Exercise 3

Exercise 4

Water

Calories IN	Calories OUT	Sleep

MONDAY

FOOD
Breakfast

Lunch

Snacks

Dinner

EXERCISE
Steps

Workout

Exercise 1

Exercise 2

Exercise 3

Exercise 4

Water

Calories IN	Calories OUT	Sleep

THURSDAY

FOOD
Breakfast

Lunch

Snacks

Dinner

EXERCISE
Steps

Workout

Exercise 1

Exercise 2

Exercise 3

Exercise 4

Water

Calories IN	Calories OUT	Sleep

FRIDAY

FOOD
Breakfast

Lunch

Snacks

Dinner

EXERCISE
Steps

Workout

Exercise 1

Exercise 2

Exercise 3

Exercise 4

Water

Calories IN	Calories OUT	Sleep

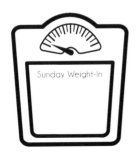

Sunday Weight-In

GOALS AND THINGS TO WORK ON THIS WEEK:

TUESDAY

FOOD

Breakfast

Lunch

Snacks

Dinner

EXERCISE

Steps

Workout

Exercise 1

Exercise 2

Exercise 3

Exercise 4

Water

Calories IN	Calories OUT	Sleep

WEDNESDAY

FOOD

Breakfast

Lunch

Snacks

Dinner

EXERCISE

Steps

Workout

Exercise 1

Exercise 2

Exercise 3

Exercise 4

Water

Calories IN	Calories OUT	Sleep

SATURDAY

FOOD

Breakfast

Lunch

Snacks

Dinner

EXERCISE

Steps

Workout

Exercise 1

Exercise 2

Exercise 3

Exercise 4

Water

Calories IN	Calories OUT	Sleep

WEEKLY SUMMARY

WORKOUTS THIS WEEK

HOW HAPPY ARE YOU WITH YOUR PROGRESS

AVERAGE WATER

Calories IN	Calories OUT	Sleep

GOALS AND THINGS TO WORK ON THIS WEEK:

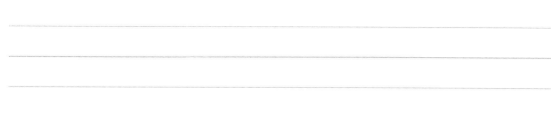

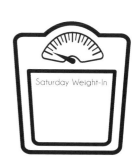

Saturday Weight-In

WEEK #31

SUNDAY

FOOD

Breakfast

Lunch

Snacks

Dinner

EXERCISE

Steps

Workout

Exercise 1

Exercise 2

Exercise 3

Exercise 4

Water

Calories IN	Calories OUT	Sleep

MONDAY

FOOD

Breakfast

Lunch

Snacks

Dinner

EXERCISE

Steps

Workout

Exercise 1

Exercise 2

Exercise 3

Exercise 4

Water

Calories IN	Calories OUT	Sleep

THURSDAY

FOOD

Breakfast

Lunch

Snacks

Dinner

EXERCISE

Steps

Workout

Exercise 1

Exercise 2

Exercise 3

Exercise 4

Water

Calories IN	Calories OUT	Sleep

FRIDAY

FOOD

Breakfast

Lunch

Snacks

Dinner

EXERCISE

Steps

Workout

Exercise 1

Exercise 2

Exercise 3

Exercise 4

Water

Calories IN	Calories OUT	Sleep

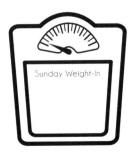

Sunday Weight-In

GOALS AND THINGS TO WORK ON THIS WEEK:

TUESDAY

FOOD

Breakfast

Lunch

Snacks

Dinner

EXERCISE

Steps

Workout

Exercise 1

Exercise 2

Exercise 3

Exercise 4

Water

Calories IN	Calories OUT	Sleep

WEDNESDAY

FOOD

Breakfast

Lunch

Snacks

Dinner

EXERCISE

Steps

Workout

Exercise 1

Exercise 2

Exercise 3

Exercise 4

Water

Calories IN	Calories OUT	Sleep

SATURDAY

FOOD

Breakfast

Lunch

Snacks

Dinner

EXERCISE

Steps

Workout

Exercise 1

Exercise 2

Exercise 3

Exercise 4

Water

Calories IN	Calories OUT	Sleep

WEEKLY SUMMARY

WORKOUTS THIS WEEK

HOW HAPPY ARE YOU WITH YOUR PROGRESS

AVERAGE WATER

Calories IN	Calories OUT	Sleep

GOALS AND THINGS TO WORK ON THIS WEEK:

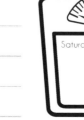

Saturday Weight-In

WEEK #32

SUNDAY

FOOD
Breakfast

Lunch

Snacks

Dinner

EXERCISE
Steps

Workout

Exercise 1

Exercise 2

Exercise 3

Exercise 4

Water

Calories IN	Calories OUT	Sleep

MONDAY

FOOD
Breakfast

Lunch

Snacks

Dinner

EXERCISE
Steps

Workout

Exercise 1

Exercise 2

Exercise 3

Exercise 4

Water

Calories IN	Calories OUT	Sleep

THURSDAY

FOOD
Breakfast

Lunch

Snacks

Dinner

EXERCISE
Steps

Workout

Exercise 1

Exercise 2

Exercise 3

Exercise 4

Water

Calories IN	Calories OUT	Sleep

FRIDAY

FOOD
Breakfast

Lunch

Snacks

Dinner

EXERCISE
Steps

Workout

Exercise 1

Exercise 2

Exercise 3

Exercise 4

Water

Calories IN	Calories OUT	Sleep

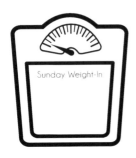

Sunday Weight-In

GOALS AND THINGS TO WORK ON THIS WEEK:

TUESDAY

FOOD

Breakfast

Lunch

Snacks

Dinner

EXERCISE

Steps

Workout

Exercise 1

Exercise 2

Exercise 3

Exercise 4

Water

Calories IN	Calories OUT	Sleep

WEDNESDAY

FOOD

Breakfast

Lunch

Snacks

Dinner

EXERCISE

Steps

Workout

Exercise 1

Exercise 2

Exercise 3

Exercise 4

Water

Calories IN	Calories OUT	Sleep

SATURDAY

FOOD

Breakfast

Lunch

Snacks

Dinner

EXERCISE

Steps

Workout

Exercise 1

Exercise 2

Exercise 3

Exercise 4

Water

Calories IN	Calories OUT	Sleep

WEEKLY SUMMARY

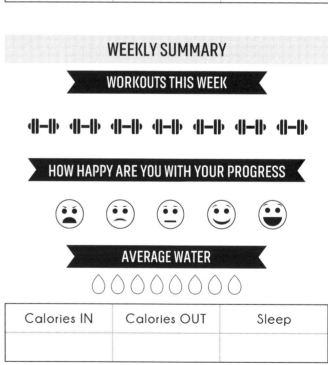

WORKOUTS THIS WEEK

HOW HAPPY ARE YOU WITH YOUR PROGRESS

AVERAGE WATER

Calories IN	Calories OUT	Sleep

GOALS AND THINGS TO WORK ON THIS WEEK:

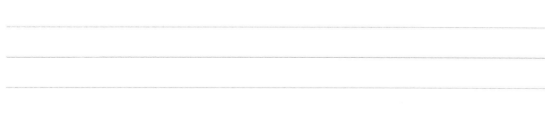

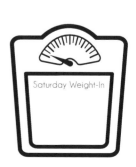

Saturday Weight-In

WEEK #33

SUNDAY

FOOD
Breakfast

Lunch

Snacks

Dinner

EXERCISE
Steps

Workout

Exercise 1

Exercise 2

Exercise 3

Exercise 4

Water

Calories IN	Calories OUT	Sleep

MONDAY

FOOD
Breakfast

Lunch

Snacks

Dinner

EXERCISE
Steps

Workout

Exercise 1

Exercise 2

Exercise 3

Exercise 4

Water

Calories IN	Calories OUT	Sleep

THURSDAY

FOOD
Breakfast

Lunch

Snacks

Dinner

EXERCISE
Steps

Workout

Exercise 1

Exercise 2

Exercise 3

Exercise 4

Water

Calories IN	Calories OUT	Sleep

FRIDAY

FOOD
Breakfast

Lunch

Snacks

Dinner

EXERCISE
Steps

Workout

Exercise 1

Exercise 2

Exercise 3

Exercise 4

Water

Calories IN	Calories OUT	Sleep

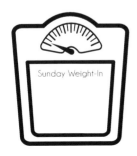

Sunday Weight-In

GOALS AND THINGS TO WORK ON THIS WEEK:

TUESDAY

FOOD

Breakfast

Lunch

Snacks

Dinner

EXERCISE

Steps

Workout

Exercise 1

Exercise 2

Exercise 3

Exercise 4

Water

Calories IN	Calories OUT	Sleep

WEDNESDAY

FOOD

Breakfast

Lunch

Snacks

Dinner

EXERCISE

Steps

Workout

Exercise 1

Exercise 2

Exercise 3

Exercise 4

Water

Calories IN	Calories OUT	Sleep

SATURDAY

FOOD

Breakfast

Lunch

Snacks

Dinner

EXERCISE

Steps

Workout

Exercise 1

Exercise 2

Exercise 3

Exercise 4

Water

Calories IN	Calories OUT	Sleep

WEEKLY SUMMARY

WORKOUTS THIS WEEK

HOW HAPPY ARE YOU WITH YOUR PROGRESS

AVERAGE WATER

Calories IN	Calories OUT	Sleep

GOALS AND THINGS TO WORK ON THIS WEEK:

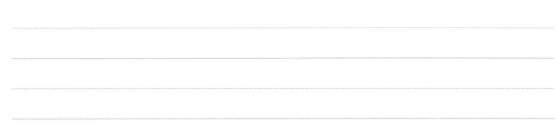

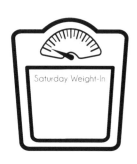

Saturday Weight-In

WEEK #34

SUNDAY

FOOD
Breakfast

Lunch

Snacks

Dinner

EXERCISE
Steps

Workout

Exercise 1

Exercise 2

Exercise 3

Exercise 4

Water

Calories IN	Calories OUT	Sleep

MONDAY

FOOD
Breakfast

Lunch

Snacks

Dinner

EXERCISE
Steps

Workout

Exercise 1

Exercise 2

Exercise 3

Exercise 4

Water

Calories IN	Calories OUT	Sleep

THURSDAY

FOOD
Breakfast

Lunch

Snacks

Dinner

EXERCISE
Steps

Workout

Exercise 1

Exercise 2

Exercise 3

Exercise 4

Water

Calories IN	Calories OUT	Sleep

FRIDAY

FOOD
Breakfast

Lunch

Snacks

Dinner

EXERCISE
Steps

Workout

Exercise 1

Exercise 2

Exercise 3

Exercise 4

Water

Calories IN	Calories OUT	Sleep

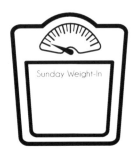

Sunday Weight-In

GOALS AND THINGS TO WORK ON THIS WEEK:

TUESDAY

FOOD

Breakfast

Lunch

Snacks

Dinner

EXERCISE

Steps

Workout

Exercise 1

Exercise 2

Exercise 3

Exercise 4

Water

Calories IN	Calories OUT	Sleep

WEDNESDAY

FOOD

Breakfast

Lunch

Snacks

Dinner

EXERCISE

Steps

Workout

Exercise 1

Exercise 2

Exercise 3

Exercise 4

Water

Calories IN	Calories OUT	Sleep

SATURDAY

FOOD

Breakfast

Lunch

Snacks

Dinner

EXERCISE

Steps

Workout

Exercise 1

Exercise 2

Exercise 3

Exercise 4

Water

Calories IN	Calories OUT	Sleep

WEEKLY SUMMARY

WORKOUTS THIS WEEK

HOW HAPPY ARE YOU WITH YOUR PROGRESS

AVERAGE WATER

Calories IN	Calories OUT	Sleep

GOALS AND THINGS TO WORK ON THIS WEEK:

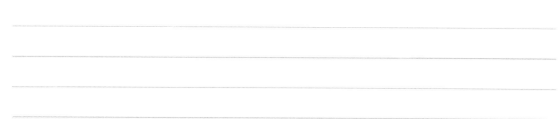

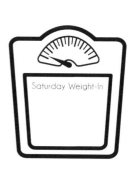

Saturday Weight-In

WEEK #35

SUNDAY

FOOD
Breakfast

Lunch

Snacks

Dinner

EXERCISE
Steps

Workout

Exercise 1

Exercise 2

Exercise 3

Exercise 4

Water

Calories IN	Calories OUT	Sleep

MONDAY

FOOD
Breakfast

Lunch

Snacks

Dinner

EXERCISE
Steps

Workout

Exercise 1

Exercise 2

Exercise 3

Exercise 4

Water

Calories IN	Calories OUT	Sleep

THURSDAY

FOOD
Breakfast

Lunch

Snacks

Dinner

EXERCISE
Steps

Workout

Exercise 1

Exercise 2

Exercise 3

Exercise 4

Water

Calories IN	Calories OUT	Sleep

FRIDAY

FOOD
Breakfast

Lunch

Snacks

Dinner

EXERCISE
Steps

Workout

Exercise 1

Exercise 2

Exercise 3

Exercise 4

Water

Calories IN	Calories OUT	Sleep

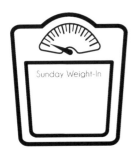

Sunday Weight-In

GOALS AND THINGS TO WORK ON THIS WEEK:

TUESDAY

FOOD

Breakfast

Lunch

Snacks

Dinner

EXERCISE

Steps

Workout

Exercise 1

Exercise 2

Exercise 3

Exercise 4

Water

Calories IN	Calories OUT	Sleep

WEDNESDAY

FOOD

Breakfast

Lunch

Snacks

Dinner

EXERCISE

Steps

Workout

Exercise 1

Exercise 2

Exercise 3

Exercise 4

Water

Calories IN	Calories OUT	Sleep

SATURDAY

FOOD

Breakfast

Lunch

Snacks

Dinner

EXERCISE

Steps

Workout

Exercise 1

Exercise 2

Exercise 3

Exercise 4

Water

Calories IN	Calories OUT	Sleep

WEEKLY SUMMARY

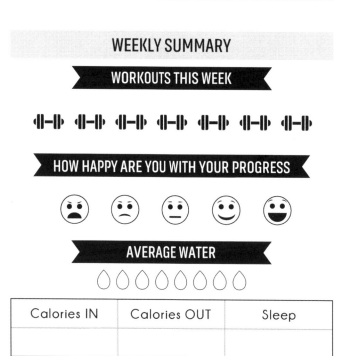

WORKOUTS THIS WEEK

HOW HAPPY ARE YOU WITH YOUR PROGRESS

AVERAGE WATER

Calories IN	Calories OUT	Sleep

GOALS AND THINGS TO WORK ON THIS WEEK:

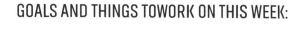

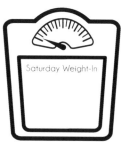

Saturday Weight-In

WEEK #36

SUNDAY

FOOD

Breakfast

Lunch

Snacks

Dinner

EXERCISE

Steps

Workout

Exercise 1

Exercise 2

Exercise 3

Exercise 4

Water

Calories IN	Calories OUT	Sleep

MONDAY

FOOD

Breakfast

Lunch

Snacks

Dinner

EXERCISE

Steps

Workout

Exercise 1

Exercise 2

Exercise 3

Exercise 4

Water

Calories IN	Calories OUT	Sleep

THURSDAY

FOOD

Breakfast

Lunch

Snacks

Dinner

EXERCISE

Steps

Workout

Exercise 1

Exercise 2

Exercise 3

Exercise 4

Water

Calories IN	Calories OUT	Sleep

FRIDAY

FOOD

Breakfast

Lunch

Snacks

Dinner

EXERCISE

Steps

Workout

Exercise 1

Exercise 2

Exercise 3

Exercise 4

Water

Calories IN	Calories OUT	Sleep

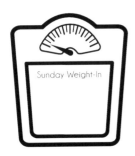

Sunday Weight-In

GOALS AND THINGS TO WORK ON THIS WEEK:

TUESDAY

FOOD

Breakfast

Lunch

Snacks

Dinner

EXERCISE

Steps

Workout

Exercise 1

Exercise 2

Exercise 3

Exercise 4

Water

Calories IN	Calories OUT	Sleep

WEDNESDAY

FOOD

Breakfast

Lunch

Snacks

Dinner

EXERCISE

Steps

Workout

Exercise 1

Exercise 2

Exercise 3

Exercise 4

Water

Calories IN	Calories OUT	Sleep

SATURDAY

FOOD

Breakfast

Lunch

Snacks

Dinner

EXERCISE

Steps

Workout

Exercise 1

Exercise 2

Exercise 3

Exercise 4

Water

Calories IN	Calories OUT	Sleep

WEEKLY SUMMARY

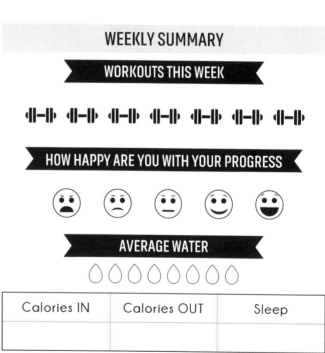

WORKOUTS THIS WEEK

HOW HAPPY ARE YOU WITH YOUR PROGRESS

AVERAGE WATER

Calories IN	Calories OUT	Sleep

GOALS AND THINGS TO WORK ON THIS WEEK:

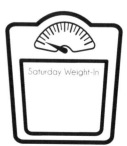

Saturday Weight-In

WEEK #37

SUNDAY

FOOD
Breakfast

Lunch

Snacks

Dinner

EXERCISE
Steps

Workout

Exercise 1

Exercise 2

Exercise 3

Exercise 4

Water

Calories IN	Calories OUT	Sleep

MONDAY

FOOD
Breakfast

Lunch

Snacks

Dinner

EXERCISE
Steps

Workout

Exercise 1

Exercise 2

Exercise 3

Exercise 4

Water

Calories IN	Calories OUT	Sleep

THURSDAY

FOOD
Breakfast

Lunch

Snacks

Dinner

EXERCISE
Steps

Workout

Exercise 1

Exercise 2

Exercise 3

Exercise 4

Water

Calories IN	Calories OUT	Sleep

FRIDAY

FOOD
Breakfast

Lunch

Snacks

Dinner

EXERCISE
Steps

Workout

Exercise 1

Exercise 2

Exercise 3

Exercise 4

Water

Calories IN	Calories OUT	Sleep

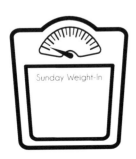

Sunday Weight-In

GOALS AND THINGS TO WORK ON THIS WEEK:

TUESDAY

FOOD

Breakfast

Lunch

Snacks

Dinner

EXERCISE

Steps

Workout

Exercise 1

Exercise 2

Exercise 3

Exercise 4

Water

Calories IN	Calories OUT	Sleep

WEDNESDAY

FOOD

Breakfast

Lunch

Snacks

Dinner

EXERCISE

Steps

Workout

Exercise 1

Exercise 2

Exercise 3

Exercise 4

Water

Calories IN	Calories OUT	Sleep

SATURDAY

FOOD

Breakfast

Lunch

Snacks

Dinner

EXERCISE

Steps

Workout

Exercise 1

Exercise 2

Exercise 3

Exercise 4

Water

Calories IN	Calories OUT	Sleep

WEEKLY SUMMARY

WORKOUTS THIS WEEK

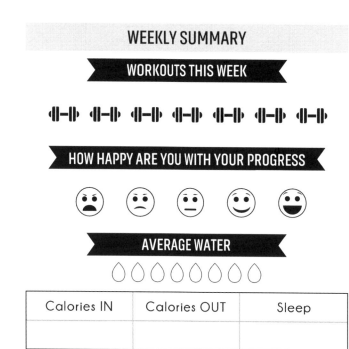

HOW HAPPY ARE YOU WITH YOUR PROGRESS

AVERAGE WATER

Calories IN	Calories OUT	Sleep

GOALS AND THINGS TO WORK ON THIS WEEK:

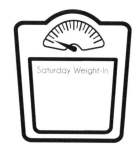

Saturday Weight-In

WEEK #38

SUNDAY

FOOD
Breakfast

Lunch

Snacks

Dinner

EXERCISE
Steps

Workout

Exercise 1

Exercise 2

Exercise 3

Exercise 4

Water

Calories IN	Calories OUT	Sleep

MONDAY

FOOD
Breakfast

Lunch

Snacks

Dinner

EXERCISE
Steps

Workout

Exercise 1

Exercise 2

Exercise 3

Exercise 4

Water

Calories IN	Calories OUT	Sleep

THURSDAY

FOOD
Breakfast

Lunch

Snacks

Dinner

EXERCISE
Steps

Workout

Exercise 1

Exercise 2

Exercise 3

Exercise 4

Water

Calories IN	Calories OUT	Sleep

FRIDAY

FOOD
Breakfast

Lunch

Snacks

Dinner

EXERCISE
Steps

Workout

Exercise 1

Exercise 2

Exercise 3

Exercise 4

Water

Calories IN	Calories OUT	Sleep

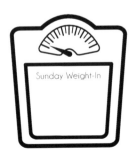

Sunday Weight-In

GOALS AND THINGS TO WORK ON THIS WEEK:

TUESDAY

FOOD

Breakfast

Lunch

Snacks

Dinner

EXERCISE

Steps

Workout

Exercise 1

Exercise 2

Exercise 3

Exercise 4

Water

Calories IN	Calories OUT	Sleep

WEDNESDAY

FOOD

Breakfast

Lunch

Snacks

Dinner

EXERCISE

Steps

Workout

Exercise 1

Exercise 2

Exercise 3

Exercise 4

Water

Calories IN	Calories OUT	Sleep

SATURDAY

FOOD

Breakfast

Lunch

Snacks

Dinner

EXERCISE

Steps

Workout

Exercise 1

Exercise 2

Exercise 3

Exercise 4

Water

Calories IN	Calories OUT	Sleep

WEEKLY SUMMARY

WORKOUTS THIS WEEK

HOW HAPPY ARE YOU WITH YOUR PROGRESS

AVERAGE WATER

Calories IN	Calories OUT	Sleep

GOALS AND THINGS TO WORK ON THIS WEEK:

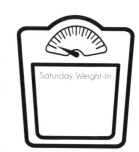

Saturday Weight-In

WEEK #39

SUNDAY

FOOD
Breakfast

Lunch

Snacks

Dinner

EXERCISE
Steps

Workout

Exercise 1

Exercise 2

Exercise 3

Exercise 4

Water

Calories IN	Calories OUT	Sleep

MONDAY

FOOD
Breakfast

Lunch

Snacks

Dinner

EXERCISE
Steps

Workout

Exercise 1

Exercise 2

Exercise 3

Exercise 4

Water

Calories IN	Calories OUT	Sleep

THURSDAY

FOOD
Breakfast

Lunch

Snacks

Dinner

EXERCISE
Steps

Workout

Exercise 1

Exercise 2

Exercise 3

Exercise 4

Water

Calories IN	Calories OUT	Sleep

FRIDAY

FOOD
Breakfast

Lunch

Snacks

Dinner

EXERCISE
Steps

Workout

Exercise 1

Exercise 2

Exercise 3

Exercise 4

Water

Calories IN	Calories OUT	Sleep

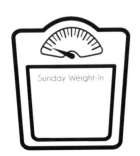

Sunday Weight-In

GOALS AND THINGS TO WORK ON THIS WEEK:

TUESDAY

FOOD

Breakfast

Lunch

Snacks

Dinner

EXERCISE

Steps

Workout

Exercise 1

Exercise 2

Exercise 3

Exercise 4

Water

Calories IN	Calories OUT	Sleep

WEDNESDAY

FOOD

Breakfast

Lunch

Snacks

Dinner

EXERCISE

Steps

Workout

Exercise 1

Exercise 2

Exercise 3

Exercise 4

Water

Calories IN	Calories OUT	Sleep

SATURDAY

FOOD

Breakfast

Lunch

Snacks

Dinner

EXERCISE

Steps

Workout

Exercise 1

Exercise 2

Exercise 3

Exercise 4

Water

Calories IN	Calories OUT	Sleep

WEEKLY SUMMARY

WORKOUTS THIS WEEK

HOW HAPPY ARE YOU WITH YOUR PROGRESS

AVERAGE WATER

Calories IN	Calories OUT	Sleep

GOALS AND THINGS TO WORK ON THIS WEEK:

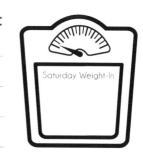

Saturday Weight-In

WEEK #40

SUNDAY

FOOD

Breakfast

Lunch

Snacks

Dinner

EXERCISE

Steps

Workout

Exercise 1

Exercise 2

Exercise 3

Exercise 4

Water

Calories IN	Calories OUT	Sleep

MONDAY

FOOD

Breakfast

Lunch

Snacks

Dinner

EXERCISE

Steps

Workout

Exercise 1

Exercise 2

Exercise 3

Exercise 4

Water

Calories IN	Calories OUT	Sleep

THURSDAY

FOOD

Breakfast

Lunch

Snacks

Dinner

EXERCISE

Steps

Workout

Exercise 1

Exercise 2

Exercise 3

Exercise 4

Water

Calories IN	Calories OUT	Sleep

FRIDAY

FOOD

Breakfast

Lunch

Snacks

Dinner

EXERCISE

Steps

Workout

Exercise 1

Exercise 2

Exercise 3

Exercise 4

Water

Calories IN	Calories OUT	Sleep

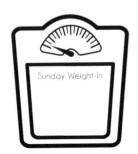

Sunday Weight-In

GOALS AND THINGS TO WORK ON THIS WEEK:

TUESDAY

FOOD

Breakfast

Lunch

Snacks

Dinner

EXERCISE

Steps

Workout

Exercise 1

Exercise 2

Exercise 3

Exercise 4

Water

Calories IN	Calories OUT	Sleep

WEDNESDAY

FOOD

Breakfast

Lunch

Snacks

Dinner

EXERCISE

Steps

Workout

Exercise 1

Exercise 2

Exercise 3

Exercise 4

Water

Calories IN	Calories OUT	Sleep

SATURDAY

FOOD

Breakfast

Lunch

Snacks

Dinner

EXERCISE

Steps

Workout

Exercise 1

Exercise 2

Exercise 3

Exercise 4

Water

Calories IN	Calories OUT	Sleep

WEEKLY SUMMARY

WORKOUTS THIS WEEK

HOW HAPPY ARE YOU WITH YOUR PROGRESS

AVERAGE WATER

Calories IN	Calories OUT	Sleep

GOALS AND THINGS TO WORK ON THIS WEEK:

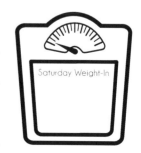

Saturday Weight-In

WEEK #41

SUNDAY

FOOD
Breakfast

Lunch

Snacks

Dinner

EXERCISE
Steps

Workout

Exercise 1

Exercise 2

Exercise 3

Exercise 4

Water

Calories IN	Calories OUT	Sleep

MONDAY

FOOD
Breakfast

Lunch

Snacks

Dinner

EXERCISE
Steps

Workout

Exercise 1

Exercise 2

Exercise 3

Exercise 4

Water

Calories IN	Calories OUT	Sleep

THURSDAY

FOOD
Breakfast

Lunch

Snacks

Dinner

EXERCISE
Steps

Workout

Exercise 1

Exercise 2

Exercise 3

Exercise 4

Water

Calories IN	Calories OUT	Sleep

FRIDAY

FOOD
Breakfast

Lunch

Snacks

Dinner

EXERCISE
Steps

Workout

Exercise 1

Exercise 2

Exercise 3

Exercise 4

Water

Calories IN	Calories OUT	Sleep

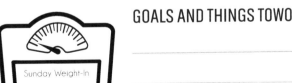

Sunday Weight-In

GOALS AND THINGS TO WORK ON THIS WEEK:

TUESDAY

FOOD

Breakfast

Lunch

Snacks

Dinner

EXERCISE

Steps

Workout

Exercise 1

Exercise 2

Exercise 3

Exercise 4

Water

Calories IN	Calories OUT	Sleep

WEDNESDAY

FOOD

Breakfast

Lunch

Snacks

Dinner

EXERCISE

Steps

Workout

Exercise 1

Exercise 2

Exercise 3

Exercise 4

Water

Calories IN	Calories OUT	Sleep

SATURDAY

FOOD

Breakfast

Lunch

Snacks

Dinner

EXERCISE

Steps

Workout

Exercise 1

Exercise 2

Exercise 3

Exercise 4

Water

Calories IN	Calories OUT	Sleep

WEEKLY SUMMARY

WORKOUTS THIS WEEK

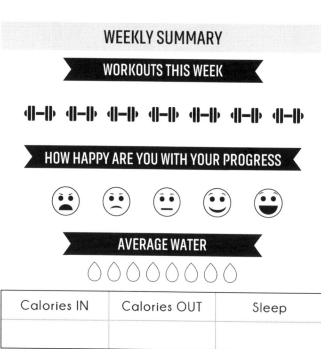

HOW HAPPY ARE YOU WITH YOUR PROGRESS

AVERAGE WATER

Calories IN	Calories OUT	Sleep

GOALS AND THINGS TOWORK ON THIS WEEK:

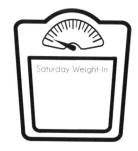

Saturday Weight-In

WEEK #42

SUNDAY

FOOD

Breakfast

Lunch

Snacks

Dinner

EXERCISE

Steps

Workout

Exercise 1

Exercise 2

Exercise 3

Exercise 4

Water

Calories IN	Calories OUT	Sleep

MONDAY

FOOD

Breakfast

Lunch

Snacks

Dinner

EXERCISE

Steps

Workout

Exercise 1

Exercise 2

Exercise 3

Exercise 4

Water

Calories IN	Calories OUT	Sleep

THURSDAY

FOOD

Breakfast

Lunch

Snacks

Dinner

EXERCISE

Steps

Workout

Exercise 1

Exercise 2

Exercise 3

Exercise 4

Water

Calories IN	Calories OUT	Sleep

FRIDAY

FOOD

Breakfast

Lunch

Snacks

Dinner

EXERCISE

Steps

Workout

Exercise 1

Exercise 2

Exercise 3

Exercise 4

Water

Calories IN	Calories OUT	Sleep

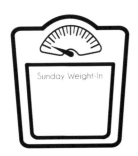

Sunday Weight-In

GOALS AND THINGS TO WORK ON THIS WEEK:

TUESDAY

FOOD

Breakfast

Lunch

Snacks

Dinner

EXERCISE

Steps

Workout

Exercise 1

Exercise 2

Exercise 3

Exercise 4

Water

Calories IN	Calories OUT	Sleep

WEDNESDAY

FOOD

Breakfast

Lunch

Snacks

Dinner

EXERCISE

Steps

Workout

Exercise 1

Exercise 2

Exercise 3

Exercise 4

Water

Calories IN	Calories OUT	Sleep

SATURDAY

FOOD

Breakfast

Lunch

Snacks

Dinner

EXERCISE

Steps

Workout

Exercise 1

Exercise 2

Exercise 3

Exercise 4

Water

Calories IN	Calories OUT	Sleep

WEEKLY SUMMARY

WORKOUTS THIS WEEK

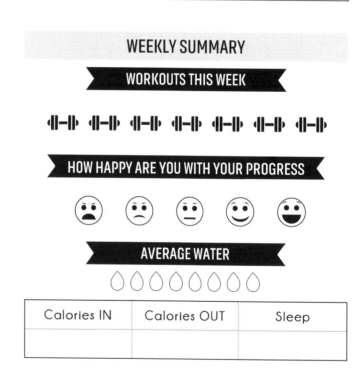

HOW HAPPY ARE YOU WITH YOUR PROGRESS

AVERAGE WATER

Calories IN	Calories OUT	Sleep

GOALS AND THINGS TO WORK ON THIS WEEK:

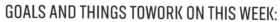

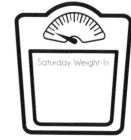

Saturday Weight-In

WEEK #43

SUNDAY

FOOD
Breakfast

Lunch

Snacks

Dinner

EXERCISE
Steps

Workout

Exercise 1

Exercise 2

Exercise 3

Exercise 4

Water

Calories IN	Calories OUT	Sleep

MONDAY

FOOD
Breakfast

Lunch

Snacks

Dinner

EXERCISE
Steps

Workout

Exercise 1

Exercise 2

Exercise 3

Exercise 4

Water

Calories IN	Calories OUT	Sleep

THURSDAY

FOOD
Breakfast

Lunch

Snacks

Dinner

EXERCISE
Steps

Workout

Exercise 1

Exercise 2

Exercise 3

Exercise 4

Water

Calories IN	Calories OUT	Sleep

FRIDAY

FOOD
Breakfast

Lunch

Snacks

Dinner

EXERCISE
Steps

Workout

Exercise 1

Exercise 2

Exercise 3

Exercise 4

Water

Calories IN	Calories OUT	Sleep

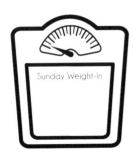
Sunday Weight-In

GOALS AND THINGS TO WORK ON THIS WEEK:

TUESDAY

FOOD

Breakfast

Lunch

Snacks

Dinner

EXERCISE

Steps

Workout

Exercise 1

Exercise 2

Exercise 3

Exercise 4

Water

Calories IN	Calories OUT	Sleep

WEDNESDAY

FOOD

Breakfast

Lunch

Snacks

Dinner

EXERCISE

Steps

Workout

Exercise 1

Exercise 2

Exercise 3

Exercise 4

Water

Calories IN	Calories OUT	Sleep

SATURDAY

FOOD

Breakfast

Lunch

Snacks

Dinner

EXERCISE

Steps

Workout

Exercise 1

Exercise 2

Exercise 3

Exercise 4

Water

Calories IN	Calories OUT	Sleep

WEEKLY SUMMARY

WORKOUTS THIS WEEK

HOW HAPPY ARE YOU WITH YOUR PROGRESS

AVERAGE WATER

Calories IN	Calories OUT	Sleep

GOALS AND THINGS TO WORK ON THIS WEEK:

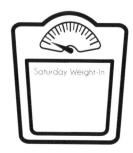

Saturday Weigh-In

WEEK #44

SUNDAY

FOOD

Breakfast

Lunch

Snacks

Dinner

EXERCISE

Steps

Workout

Exercise 1

Exercise 2

Exercise 3

Exercise 4

Water

Calories IN	Calories OUT	Sleep

MONDAY

FOOD

Breakfast

Lunch

Snacks

Dinner

EXERCISE

Steps

Workout

Exercise 1

Exercise 2

Exercise 3

Exercise 4

Water

Calories IN	Calories OUT	Sleep

THURSDAY

FOOD

Breakfast

Lunch

Snacks

Dinner

EXERCISE

Steps

Workout

Exercise 1

Exercise 2

Exercise 3

Exercise 4

Water

Calories IN	Calories OUT	Sleep

FRIDAY

FOOD

Breakfast

Lunch

Snacks

Dinner

EXERCISE

Steps

Workout

Exercise 1

Exercise 2

Exercise 3

Exercise 4

Water

Calories IN	Calories OUT	Sleep

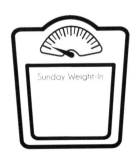

Sunday Weight-In

GOALS AND THINGS TO WORK ON THIS WEEK:

TUESDAY

FOOD

Breakfast

Lunch

Snacks

Dinner

EXERCISE

Steps

Workout

Exercise 1

Exercise 2

Exercise 3

Exercise 4

Water

Calories IN	Calories OUT	Sleep

WEDNESDAY

FOOD

Breakfast

Lunch

Snacks

Dinner

EXERCISE

Steps

Workout

Exercise 1

Exercise 2

Exercise 3

Exercise 4

Water

Calories IN	Calories OUT	Sleep

SATURDAY

FOOD

Breakfast

Lunch

Snacks

Dinner

EXERCISE

Steps

Workout

Exercise 1

Exercise 2

Exercise 3

Exercise 4

Water

Calories IN	Calories OUT	Sleep

WEEKLY SUMMARY

WORKOUTS THIS WEEK

HOW HAPPY ARE YOU WITH YOUR PROGRESS

AVERAGE WATER

Calories IN	Calories OUT	Sleep

GOALS AND THINGS TO WORK ON THIS WEEK:

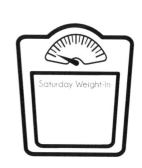

Saturday Weight-In

WEEK #45

SUNDAY

FOOD
Breakfast

Lunch

Snacks

Dinner

EXERCISE
Steps

Workout

Exercise 1

Exercise 2

Exercise 3

Exercise 4

Water

Calories IN	Calories OUT	Sleep

MONDAY

FOOD
Breakfast

Lunch

Snacks

Dinner

EXERCISE
Steps

Workout

Exercise 1

Exercise 2

Exercise 3

Exercise 4

Water

Calories IN	Calories OUT	Sleep

THURSDAY

FOOD
Breakfast

Lunch

Snacks

Dinner

EXERCISE
Steps

Workout

Exercise 1

Exercise 2

Exercise 3

Exercise 4

Water

Calories IN	Calories OUT	Sleep

FRIDAY

FOOD
Breakfast

Lunch

Snacks

Dinner

EXERCISE
Steps

Workout

Exercise 1

Exercise 2

Exercise 3

Exercise 4

Water

Calories IN	Calories OUT	Sleep

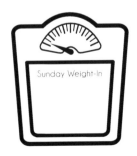

Sunday Weight-In

GOALS AND THINGS TO WORK ON THIS WEEK:

TUESDAY

FOOD

Breakfast

Lunch

Snacks

Dinner

EXERCISE

Steps

Workout

Exercise 1

Exercise 2

Exercise 3

Exercise 4

Water

Calories IN	Calories OUT	Sleep

WEDNESDAY

FOOD

Breakfast

Lunch

Snacks

Dinner

EXERCISE

Steps

Workout

Exercise 1

Exercise 2

Exercise 3

Exercise 4

Water

Calories IN	Calories OUT	Sleep

SATURDAY

FOOD

Breakfast

Lunch

Snacks

Dinner

EXERCISE

Steps

Workout

Exercise 1

Exercise 2

Exercise 3

Exercise 4

Water

Calories IN	Calories OUT	Sleep

WEEKLY SUMMARY

WORKOUTS THIS WEEK

HOW HAPPY ARE YOU WITH YOUR PROGRESS

AVERAGE WATER

Calories IN	Calories OUT	Sleep

GOALS AND THINGS TO WORK ON THIS WEEK:

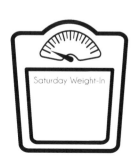

Saturday Weight-In

WEEK #46

SUNDAY

FOOD

Breakfast

Lunch

Snacks

Dinner

EXERCISE

Steps

Workout

Exercise 1

Exercise 2

Exercise 3

Exercise 4

Water

Calories IN	Calories OUT	Sleep

MONDAY

FOOD

Breakfast

Lunch

Snacks

Dinner

EXERCISE

Steps

Workout

Exercise 1

Exercise 2

Exercise 3

Exercise 4

Water

Calories IN	Calories OUT	Sleep

THURSDAY

FOOD

Breakfast

Lunch

Snacks

Dinner

EXERCISE

Steps

Workout

Exercise 1

Exercise 2

Exercise 3

Exercise 4

Water

Calories IN	Calories OUT	Sleep

FRIDAY

FOOD

Breakfast

Lunch

Snacks

Dinner

EXERCISE

Steps

Workout

Exercise 1

Exercise 2

Exercise 3

Exercise 4

Water

Calories IN	Calories OUT	Sleep

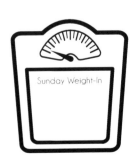

Sunday Weight-In

GOALS AND THINGS TO WORK ON THIS WEEK:

TUESDAY

FOOD

Breakfast

Lunch

Snacks

Dinner

EXERCISE

Steps

Workout

Exercise 1

Exercise 2

Exercise 3

Exercise 4

Water

Calories IN	Calories OUT	Sleep

WEDNESDAY

FOOD

Breakfast

Lunch

Snacks

Dinner

EXERCISE

Steps

Workout

Exercise 1

Exercise 2

Exercise 3

Exercise 4

Water

Calories IN	Calories OUT	Sleep

SATURDAY

FOOD

Breakfast

Lunch

Snacks

Dinner

EXERCISE

Steps

Workout

Exercise 1

Exercise 2

Exercise 3

Exercise 4

Water

Calories IN	Calories OUT	Sleep

WEEKLY SUMMARY

WORKOUTS THIS WEEK

HOW HAPPY ARE YOU WITH YOUR PROGRESS

AVERAGE WATER

Calories IN	Calories OUT	Sleep

GOALS AND THINGS TOWORK ON THIS WEEK:

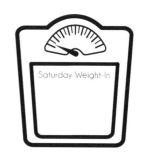

Saturday Weight-In

WEEK #47

SUNDAY

FOOD	EXERCISE
Breakfast	Steps
	Workout
Lunch	Exercise 1
	Exercise 2
Snacks	Exercise 3
	Exercise 4
Dinner	Water

Calories IN	Calories OUT	Sleep

MONDAY

FOOD	EXERCISE
Breakfast	Steps
	Workout
Lunch	Exercise 1
	Exercise 2
Snacks	Exercise 3
	Exercise 4
Dinner	Water

Calories IN	Calories OUT	Sleep

THURSDAY

FOOD	EXERCISE
Breakfast	Steps
	Workout
Lunch	Exercise 1
	Exercise 2
Snacks	Exercise 3
	Exercise 4
Dinner	Water

Calories IN	Calories OUT	Sleep

FRIDAY

FOOD	EXERCISE
Breakfast	Steps
	Workout
Lunch	Exercise 1
	Exercise 2
Snacks	Exercise 3
	Exercise 4
Dinner	Water

Calories IN	Calories OUT	Sleep

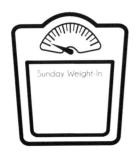

Sunday Weight-In

GOALS AND THINGS TO WORK ON THIS WEEK:

TUESDAY

FOOD

Breakfast

Lunch

Snacks

Dinner

EXERCISE

Steps

Workout

Exercise 1

Exercise 2

Exercise 3

Exercise 4

Water

Calories IN	Calories OUT	Sleep

WEDNESDAY

FOOD

Breakfast

Lunch

Snacks

Dinner

EXERCISE

Steps

Workout

Exercise 1

Exercise 2

Exercise 3

Exercise 4

Water

Calories IN	Calories OUT	Sleep

SATURDAY

FOOD

Breakfast

Lunch

Snacks

Dinner

EXERCISE

Steps

Workout

Exercise 1

Exercise 2

Exercise 3

Exercise 4

Water

Calories IN	Calories OUT	Sleep

WEEKLY SUMMARY

WORKOUTS THIS WEEK

HOW HAPPY ARE YOU WITH YOUR PROGRESS

AVERAGE WATER

Calories IN	Calories OUT	Sleep

GOALS AND THINGS TO WORK ON THIS WEEK:

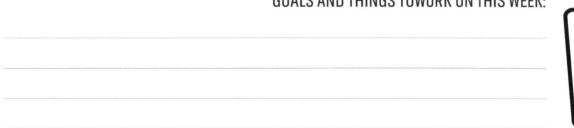

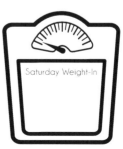

Saturday Weight-In

WEEK #48

SUNDAY

FOOD
Breakfast

Lunch

Snacks

Dinner

EXERCISE
Steps

Workout

Exercise 1

Exercise 2

Exercise 3

Exercise 4

Water

Calories IN	Calories OUT	Sleep

MONDAY

FOOD
Breakfast

Lunch

Snacks

Dinner

EXERCISE
Steps

Workout

Exercise 1

Exercise 2

Exercise 3

Exercise 4

Water

Calories IN	Calories OUT	Sleep

THURSDAY

FOOD
Breakfast

Lunch

Snacks

Dinner

EXERCISE
Steps

Workout

Exercise 1

Exercise 2

Exercise 3

Exercise 4

Water

Calories IN	Calories OUT	Sleep

FRIDAY

FOOD
Breakfast

Lunch

Snacks

Dinner

EXERCISE
Steps

Workout

Exercise 1

Exercise 2

Exercise 3

Exercise 4

Water

Calories IN	Calories OUT	Sleep

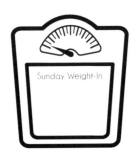
Sunday Weight-In

GOALS AND THINGS TO WORK ON THIS WEEK:

TUESDAY

FOOD

Breakfast

Lunch

Snacks

Dinner

EXERCISE

Steps

Workout

Exercise 1

Exercise 2

Exercise 3

Exercise 4

Water

Calories IN	Calories OUT	Sleep

WEDNESDAY

FOOD

Breakfast

Lunch

Snacks

Dinner

EXERCISE

Steps

Workout

Exercise 1

Exercise 2

Exercise 3

Exercise 4

Water

Calories IN	Calories OUT	Sleep

SATURDAY

FOOD

Breakfast

Lunch

Snacks

Dinner

EXERCISE

Steps

Workout

Exercise 1

Exercise 2

Exercise 3

Exercise 4

Water

Calories IN	Calories OUT	Sleep

WEEKLY SUMMARY

WORKOUTS THIS WEEK

HOW HAPPY ARE YOU WITH YOUR PROGRESS

AVERAGE WATER

Calories IN	Calories OUT	Sleep

GOALS AND THINGS TO WORK ON THIS WEEK:

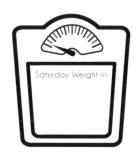

Saturday Weight-In

WEEK #49

SUNDAY

FOOD
Breakfast

Lunch

Snacks

Dinner

EXERCISE
Steps

Workout

Exercise 1

Exercise 2

Exercise 3

Exercise 4

Water

Calories IN	Calories OUT	Sleep

MONDAY

FOOD
Breakfast

Lunch

Snacks

Dinner

EXERCISE
Steps

Workout

Exercise 1

Exercise 2

Exercise 3

Exercise 4

Water

Calories IN	Calories OUT	Sleep

THURSDAY

FOOD
Breakfast

Lunch

Snacks

Dinner

EXERCISE
Steps

Workout

Exercise 1

Exercise 2

Exercise 3

Exercise 4

Water

Calories IN	Calories OUT	Sleep

FRIDAY

FOOD
Breakfast

Lunch

Snacks

Dinner

EXERCISE
Steps

Workout

Exercise 1

Exercise 2

Exercise 3

Exercise 4

Water

Calories IN	Calories OUT	Sleep

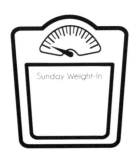

Sunday Weight-In

GOALS AND THINGS TO WORK ON THIS WEEK:

TUESDAY

FOOD

Breakfast

Lunch

Snacks

Dinner

EXERCISE

Steps

Workout

Exercise 1

Exercise 2

Exercise 3

Exercise 4

Water

Calories IN	Calories OUT	Sleep

WEDNESDAY

FOOD

Breakfast

Lunch

Snacks

Dinner

EXERCISE

Steps

Workout

Exercise 1

Exercise 2

Exercise 3

Exercise 4

Water

Calories IN	Calories OUT	Sleep

SATURDAY

FOOD

Breakfast

Lunch

Snacks

Dinner

EXERCISE

Steps

Workout

Exercise 1

Exercise 2

Exercise 3

Exercise 4

Water

Calories IN	Calories OUT	Sleep

WEEKLY SUMMARY

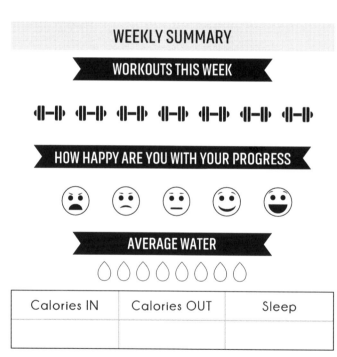

WORKOUTS THIS WEEK

HOW HAPPY ARE YOU WITH YOUR PROGRESS

AVERAGE WATER

Calories IN	Calories OUT	Sleep

GOALS AND THINGS TO WORK ON THIS WEEK:

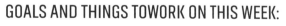

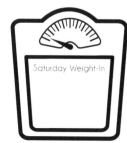

Saturday Weight-In

WEEK #50

SUNDAY

FOOD
Breakfast

Lunch

Snacks

Dinner

EXERCISE
Steps

Workout

Exercise 1

Exercise 2

Exercise 3

Exercise 4

Water

Calories IN	Calories OUT	Sleep

MONDAY

FOOD
Breakfast

Lunch

Snacks

Dinner

EXERCISE
Steps

Workout

Exercise 1

Exercise 2

Exercise 3

Exercise 4

Water

Calories IN	Calories OUT	Sleep

THURSDAY

FOOD
Breakfast

Lunch

Snacks

Dinner

EXERCISE
Steps

Workout

Exercise 1

Exercise 2

Exercise 3

Exercise 4

Water

Calories IN	Calories OUT	Sleep

FRIDAY

FOOD
Breakfast

Lunch

Snacks

Dinner

EXERCISE
Steps

Workout

Exercise 1

Exercise 2

Exercise 3

Exercise 4

Water

Calories IN	Calories OUT	Sleep

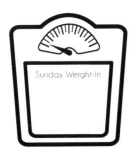

Sunday Weight-In

GOALS AND THINGS TO WORK ON THIS WEEK:

TUESDAY

FOOD

Breakfast

Lunch

Snacks

Dinner

EXERCISE

Steps

Workout

Exercise 1

Exercise 2

Exercise 3

Exercise 4

Water

Calories IN	Calories OUT	Sleep

WEDNESDAY

FOOD

Breakfast

Lunch

Snacks

Dinner

EXERCISE

Steps

Workout

Exercise 1

Exercise 2

Exercise 3

Exercise 4

Water

Calories IN	Calories OUT	Sleep

SATURDAY

FOOD

Breakfast

Lunch

Snacks

Dinner

EXERCISE

Steps

Workout

Exercise 1

Exercise 2

Exercise 3

Exercise 4

Water

Calories IN	Calories OUT	Sleep

WEEKLY SUMMARY

WORKOUTS THIS WEEK

HOW HAPPY ARE YOU WITH YOUR PROGRESS

AVERAGE WATER

Calories IN	Calories OUT	Sleep

GOALS AND THINGS TO WORK ON THIS WEEK:

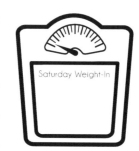

Saturday Weight-In

WEEK #51

SUNDAY

FOOD
Breakfast

Lunch

Snacks

Dinner

EXERCISE
Steps

Workout

Exercise 1

Exercise 2

Exercise 3

Exercise 4

Water

Calories IN	Calories OUT	Sleep

MONDAY

FOOD
Breakfast

Lunch

Snacks

Dinner

EXERCISE
Steps

Workout

Exercise 1

Exercise 2

Exercise 3

Exercise 4

Water

Calories IN	Calories OUT	Sleep

THURSDAY

FOOD
Breakfast

Lunch

Snacks

Dinner

EXERCISE
Steps

Workout

Exercise 1

Exercise 2

Exercise 3

Exercise 4

Water

Calories IN	Calories OUT	Sleep

FRIDAY

FOOD
Breakfast

Lunch

Snacks

Dinner

EXERCISE
Steps

Workout

Exercise 1

Exercise 2

Exercise 3

Exercise 4

Water

Calories IN	Calories OUT	Sleep

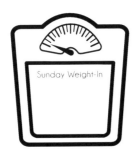

Sunday Weight-In

GOALS AND THINGS TO WORK ON THIS WEEK:

TUESDAY

FOOD

Breakfast

Lunch

Snacks

Dinner

EXERCISE

Steps

Workout

Exercise 1

Exercise 2

Exercise 3

Exercise 4

Water

Calories IN	Calories OUT	Sleep

WEDNESDAY

FOOD

Breakfast

Lunch

Snacks

Dinner

EXERCISE

Steps

Workout

Exercise 1

Exercise 2

Exercise 3

Exercise 4

Water

Calories IN	Calories OUT	Sleep

SATURDAY

FOOD

Breakfast

Lunch

Snacks

Dinner

EXERCISE

Steps

Workout

Exercise 1

Exercise 2

Exercise 3

Exercise 4

Water

Calories IN	Calories OUT	Sleep

WEEKLY SUMMARY

WORKOUTS THIS WEEK

HOW HAPPY ARE YOU WITH YOUR PROGRESS

AVERAGE WATER

Calories IN	Calories OUT	Sleep

GOALS AND THINGS TOWORK ON THIS WEEK:

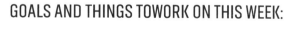

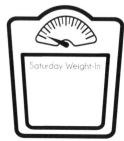

Saturday Weight-In

WEEK #52

SUNDAY

FOOD

Breakfast

Lunch

Snacks

Dinner

EXERCISE

Steps

Workout

Exercise 1

Exercise 2

Exercise 3

Exercise 4

Water

Calories IN	Calories OUT	Sleep

MONDAY

FOOD

Breakfast

Lunch

Snacks

Dinner

EXERCISE

Steps

Workout

Exercise 1

Exercise 2

Exercise 3

Exercise 4

Water

Calories IN	Calories OUT	Sleep

THURSDAY

FOOD

Breakfast

Lunch

Snacks

Dinner

EXERCISE

Steps

Workout

Exercise 1

Exercise 2

Exercise 3

Exercise 4

Water

Calories IN	Calories OUT	Sleep

FRIDAY

FOOD

Breakfast

Lunch

Snacks

Dinner

EXERCISE

Steps

Workout

Exercise 1

Exercise 2

Exercise 3

Exercise 4

Water

Calories IN	Calories OUT	Sleep

Sunday Weight-In

GOALS AND THINGS TO WORK ON THIS WEEK:

TUESDAY

FOOD

Breakfast

Lunch

Snacks

Dinner

EXERCISE

Steps

Workout

Exercise 1

Exercise 2

Exercise 3

Exercise 4

Water

Calories IN	Calories OUT	Sleep

WEDNESDAY

FOOD

Breakfast

Lunch

Snacks

Dinner

EXERCISE

Steps

Workout

Exercise 1

Exercise 2

Exercise 3

Exercise 4

Water

Calories IN	Calories OUT	Sleep

SATURDAY

FOOD

Breakfast

Lunch

Snacks

Dinner

EXERCISE

Steps

Workout

Exercise 1

Exercise 2

Exercise 3

Exercise 4

Water

Calories IN	Calories OUT	Sleep

WEEKLY SUMMARY

WORKOUTS THIS WEEK

HOW HAPPY ARE YOU WITH YOUR PROGRESS

AVERAGE WATER

Calories IN	Calories OUT	Sleep

GOALS AND THINGS TO WORK ON THIS WEEK:

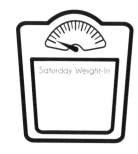

Saturday Weight-In

NOTES

NOTES

NOTES

Made in the USA
Monee, IL
22 January 2020